D1806630

KEEP FIT

KEEP FIT

Exercises
for everyone

Eileen Fowler

BOOK CLUB ASSOCIATES
LONDON

Author's acknowledgement

I am most grateful to Dr Don Anthony for the encouragement and advice he gave me during the preparation of this book.

Dr Anthony is a university and college lecturer in physical education, Director of the Centre for International Sports Exchange, a member of the National Olympic Committee, a sports consultant and well-known writer on fitness.

This edition published 1983 by Book Club Associates by arrangement with Piatkus Books

© 1983 Eileen Fowler

First published in 1983 by
Judy Piatkus (Publishers)
Limited of Loughton, Essex

British Library Cataloguing in Publication Data

Fowler, Eileen
  Keep fit.
  1. Physical fitness
  I. Title
  613.7   RA781
    ISBN 0-86188-259-8
    ISBN 0-86188-265-2 pbk

Illustrations and design by
Astrid Publishing Consultants Ltd

Typeset by Wyvern Typesetting Ltd, Bristol
Printed in Great Britain at
The Pitman Press, Bath

Contents

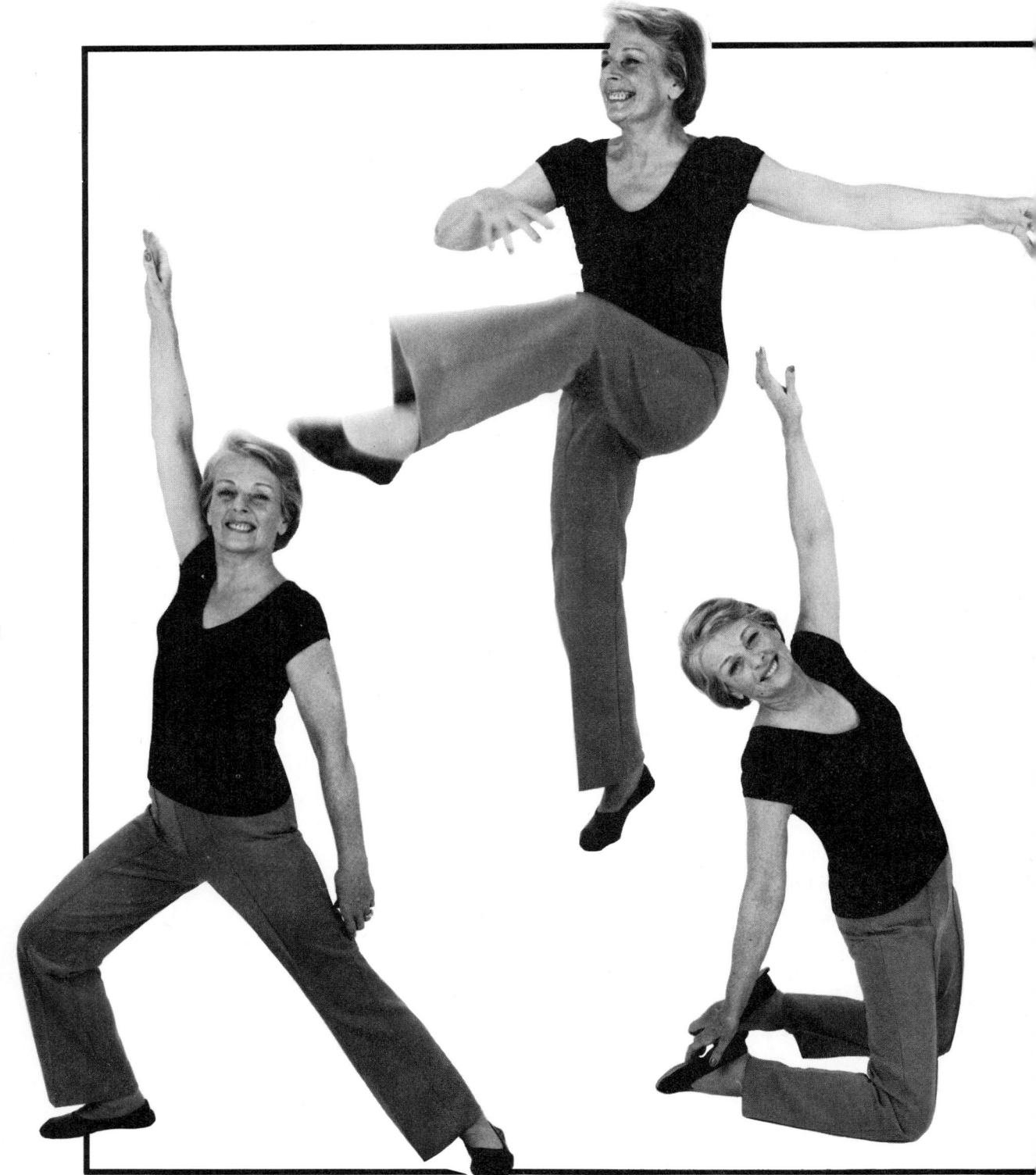

Introduction

As I am writing about the importance of keeping fit and suggesting that you might find my words of benefit, I think I should explain why I am doing this. I was born in 1906, and from the age of three I loved to move. I wanted to run, to dance, to exercise, to swim, to ride – anything that would make me move. I liked the feeling of health and fitness that exercise gave me – and I liked the relaxation that followed, the way it made me look, and my livelier brain. Of course, I didn't understand the whys and wherefores, or why not everyone felt this way.

Then, during my years in the theatre, there seemed to be no time for all this activity. I ate too much of all the wrong foods, and late nights and parties gave me indigestion. At the end of each run I would be highly strung, nervous and liverish. And in my twenties I was tired. Fortunately, I discovered a new way of living. I listened to my mother who was fit, wise and beautiful. I left the stage and started to teach keep fit. I have never looked back. Years and years of study have taught me how to live, how to keep my weight at just under $8\frac{1}{2}$ stone (at 5′ 5″), and to be able to do everything I have to do and want to do.

May I tell you about it?

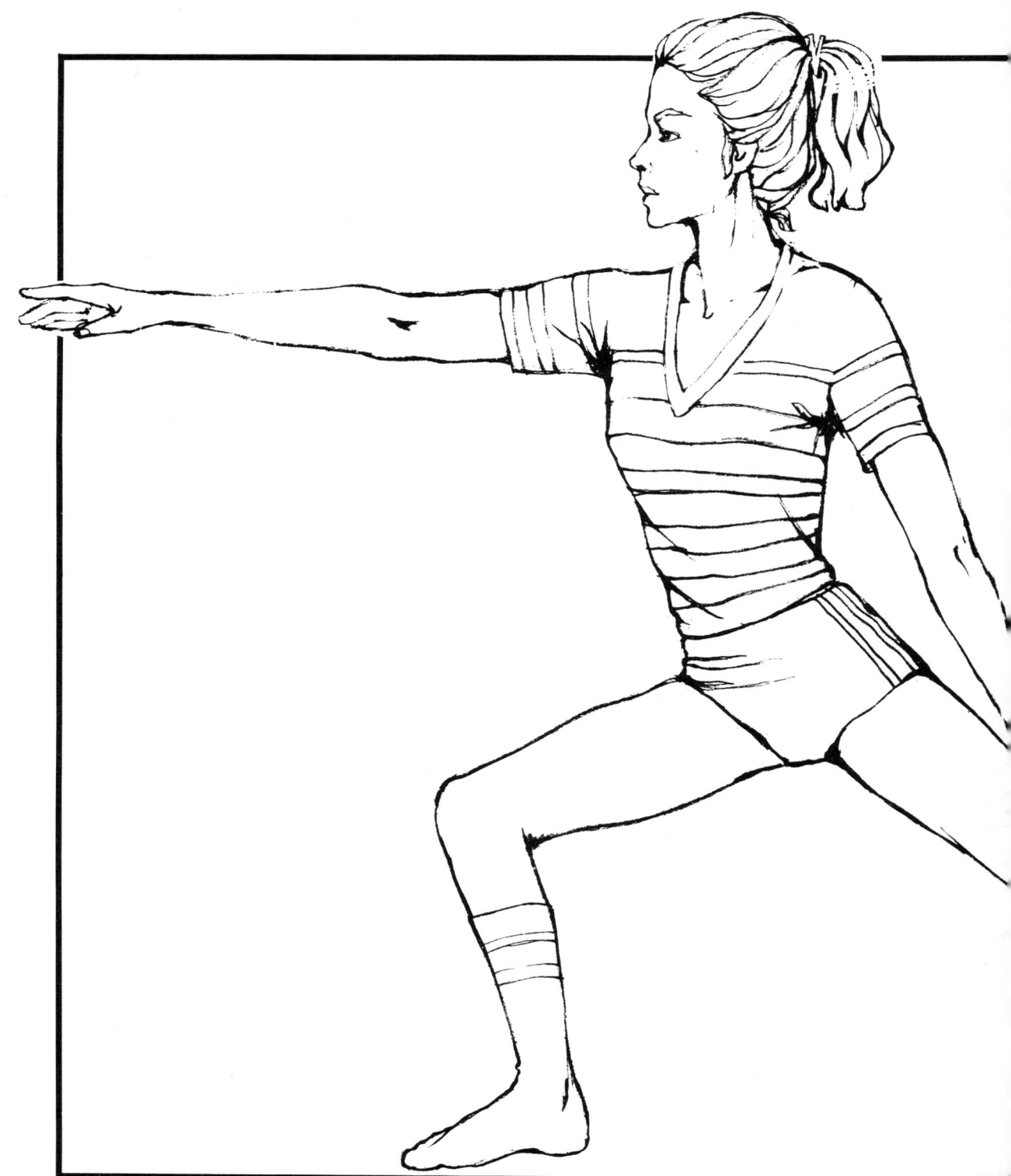

Chapter 1

The body needs activity

The diminishing desire for exercise. The dangers of inactivity. Exercise is the body's natural tonic. The need to get fit and stay fit. The six essentials for fitness and health: exercise, fresh air, active leisure, the right food, relaxation and sound sleep. Exercise is not a boring routine but a way of life which is truly valuable and quite astonishing in its results.

If you are fortunate enough to spend part of your leisure-time playing squash, tennis or rounds of golf, or perhaps sailing away at weekends, fitness is unlikely to be a problem. I am concerned with those men, women and young people who need a more simple method of keeping fit in order to counteract the effects of a sedentary way of life.

Many people are forced to be relatively inactive due to their occupation; they are obliged to sit for long hours every day working or commuting. There is the ever-present risk of delay, and the constant pressure of having to keep appointments by a clock that will not wait. Exciting and rewarding as this lifestyle may be, it often adds up to a good deal of stress and strain by the end of the day. Then there is the journey home, a meal to eat, and the armchair beckons. Perhaps we ought to go out and stretch our legs, but there is always the weekend. So we turn on the television set . . . and it becomes a habit.

It is insidious, this gradually diminishing desire for exercise. We are tired and long to relax but the armchair and television set are not always the answer. We know that we need exercise, but do we know just how important it is? Does it matter if we ignore it? Of course it does.

Exercise is the finest preventative medicine you can take. It is not just physical, it relaxes you mentally. Exercising the body leads to a more positive way of thinking; it encourages a more optimistic outlook and generates the determination to keep going. Exercise is the body's natural tonic but, like all tonics, it has to be taken at the right time. It is useless to force an exhausted body to move when it is crying out for rest; but if the exhaustion is more mental than physical, then, like the man who walks his dog or the secretary whose keep fit class banishes her weariness, exercise is the answer.

Even young people get tired. Tiredness is a chronic illness, an occupational hazard. But why? Don't we all know that the trouble is often lack of exercise? Don't we all realise that strong, toned-up muscles would make all the difference?

To counteract too much sitting, stuffy offices, crowded trains and long hours standing, we need an antidote. We may not be able to change our jobs or our surroundings but we can change ourselves. We can make ourselves so fit that the harassment can be a challenge not a killer. Fitness can become a shield, a defence against the problems that beset us. And to be really fit we need exercise. Real fitness can prevent the keen young 'whizz kid' from becoming the tired businessman, and can take him up the ladder of success without his having to resort to the crutches that are so readily available today. We too quickly resort to pep pills, something to make us sleep, or just one more drink to break the tension. Who prescribes these crutches? Very often we do ourselves, and that is why I think we should change the medicine. There are other ways, natural ways, to tackle lack of energy, anxiety and tension. Once these methods are adopted and have become a habit, we are set for life.

Let us look at, examine and accept what I consider to be the six essentials for health. These are exercise, fresh air, the right food, active leisure, relaxation and sound sleep. All six are equally important. There is no doubt that anyone of any age – male or female – who cares to follow these simple rules for healthy living will gain tremendous benefit.

Exercise

The sense of well-being promoted by exercise cannot be easily explained. It is necessary for you to feel it for yourself. To stretch and bend, twist and relax is exhilarating. We are meant to move; to warm up gently, to pep up the circulation, and to loosen up and extend our muscles and ourselves. It is good for us to stand tall and confident with no dreary slumping in the middle; to lift the chest so that there is a longer space between chest and hips. We need to be able to breathe deeply, to expand, to reach up and away, and to feel fitter every time we exercise.

Our muscles are our framework, the controlling force for what we can or cannot do, and it makes sense to look after them. If you use your muscles the right way they will let you do more and more. But if you don't keep them polished up, when you want them to work for you they will not be able to. We all know what it is like to bring into play muscles that have not been used for years, and to suffer the stiffness and pain that is caused by sudden exercise. We are meant to use our bodies to their fullest extent, and unless there is a medical reason why we should remain passive, then move we must. Muscle tone is good for the appearance both now and in later life. It ensures that the skin remains light and firm, with no loose or flabby necks, upper arms, chests, stomachs or thighs. Exercise works.

There are people who confess to hating exercise because when they were young they found it too gymnastic or preferred dancing or reading to games. We are fortunate today because there are types of movement and sport to suit everyone. The choice is wide and the standards very high. The exercises I give in Chapters 9 to 18 are designed to be of the greatest possible benefit to everyone in the family – from those members who are in their early teens to retired people in their late seventies. Today, men and women follow practically the same training routines in sport, swimming and athletics, and this rule applies to keep fit exercises too. They simply respond differently to the training, and have obvious physical differences.

Many of the exercises will strike a familiar note, but when performed with ease and relaxation the whole picture changes. Gone is any kind of jerk or military style; the movements are felt throughout the body and are flowing and satisfying. There is no fear of exhaustion because the accent is constantly changing. Each muscle group is given time to rest so that the performer is not tired at the end of a session but finishes refreshed. It is easy to feel fit if we exercise this modern fluid way, moving not just arms and legs but the whole body. Every muscle is brought into play and gradually toned and strengthened. Joints are eased and we become more mobile, more able to withstand the stresses and strains of daily life. It may be called free movement but it is strong and efficient and provides a base for other activities.

So let us look again at the word exercise and see it in its true light, not as a boring routine but as a way of life which is valuable and quite astonishing in its results.

Good posture

When you think about figure problems, they are much the same for men as for women, whether you are young, middle aged or retired. Some people stand tall throughout their lives quite naturally, but far more forget about good posture, deep breathing and the necessity to keep the head up and to hold it high. Once the head is allowed to drop forward, even a little, the shoulders follow and before long the slack neck and back muscles fail to hold the body upright, and (horror of horrors) there is a chance that a dowager's hump might develop in later life. Things can get worse. You may not only walk head first, but the weak back and stomach muscles which should work together to support your figure allow the stomach to protrude beyond the chest, instead of the other way round. Having let go to this extent, the hips are not too happy; joints tend to stiffen, steps become shorter, a stick is necessary, and feet don't like being put down in a flat manner.

Shall I go on?

I have watched the process happen many times, bit by bit, and it is quite unnecessary. We know about the law of gravity pulling us down, and many things we do causing us to bend forward or stoop. So why don't we make sure, once and for all, that it never

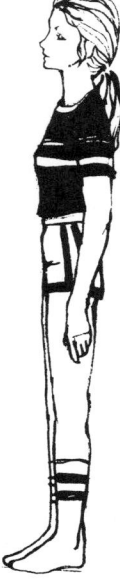

Posture test
Stand with your back to a wall and try to touch it most of the way down. Walk forward in that position.

happens to us. Use exercise to counteract the side effects of daily living. Learn to stand well and to move well.

Start with the correct way to stand. Good posture allows the body to work properly. The organs can function more easily, and certainly the lungs can do their job with greater comfort. Being able to stand up to one's full height is very important.

Find out if your head is held high and whether your shoulders are straight or rounded. Start with the Posture Test. Relax your back into the wall so that you are touching it most of the way down, remembering that the spine is curved. Flatten yourself against it as far as possible, then walk forward and away, not stiffly but quite naturally. This exercise will give you some idea of how you normally stand and walk. If you have to make any changes, check that your posture is improving by doing the posture test each day. It will only take a minute but it will remind you to stand tall.

Now for the Shoulder Test. Back to the wall and stand as before. Raise one arm forward and upward above your head and try to touch the wall with the back of your hand. If your shoulders are perfectly straight you will be able to keep your hand on the wall with the arm dead straight and close to your head. If it bends at the elbow, watch those round shoulders. Try it with the other arm. Sometimes, one arm is bent and the other straight. Practise until both arms are straight – but only one arm must go up at a time, never the two together.

Shoulder test
Back to a wall, take one arm forward and upward to lie flat against the wall close to your head. Stretch and lower. Repeat with other arm.

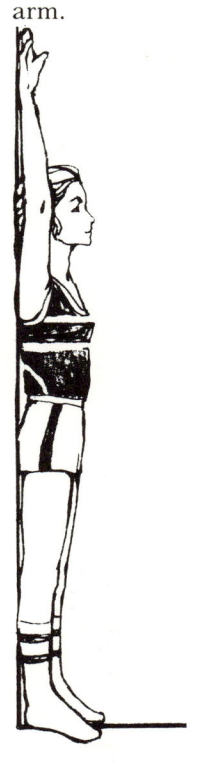

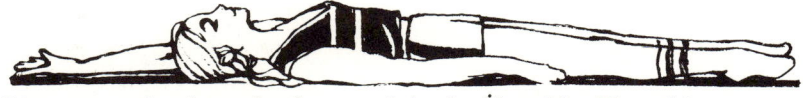

Lie on your back on the floor and do the Shoulder Test this way.

Fresh air

We all know how essential it is to get out in the fresh air, but isn't it easier sometimes to stay indoors? In the summer going out is a joy, but it's much more of an effort on cold wintry days. There is the odd outdoor job that can't wait, but it's warm and comfortable indoors . . .

Somehow, we have got to convince ourselves that it is very important to get out as often as we can. The build-up of the warmth and the dryness of artificial heat leaves us rather dehydrated if we are inside for too long. Central heating can dry up hair and complexions, and overheated rooms can actually be a health risk. It is essential to get out in the winter because the windows are not wide open and we need oxygen to cleanse the blood stream, to help us to breathe more deeply, to brighten our eyes and skin.

No time to walk? Well, forget the freezer and shop more often. Walk to work. It doesn't matter what we do or where we go, as long as we are prepared to wrap up and get out. You can't beat that fresh air look. A Scottish friend of mine used to say: 'But Eileen, the fresh air feeds me.' It's so young. How much better we all look in the summer months. It is not only the sunshine – and too much sun can age the skin – it is simply being out in the fresh air every moment you can spare. It can be windy or showery, what does it matter? I live by the sea and I watch the tired grey faces of the visitors change before my eyes as their owners stay out in the sea air until the last possible moment. Skins freshen; eyes shine; steps hasten; hair blows in the wind, full of vitality.

It is a wonderful gift, fresh sea or country air, and within the reach of most of us. It is better not to wait until holiday time, but to put these outings into your daily life. Start to cycle, play tennis or golf, walk, or even jog.

Jogging

Please be careful if you jog. Your shoes must have a well-padded heel, and special jogging shoes are available. Before starting, the not-so-young should remember that tendons and muscles which have not been used this way for years could cause a lot of problems. It is also important not to confuse jogging with sprinting. If you run on the ball of the foot you can pull the achilles tendon, which is highly dangerous and can strain calf muscles too. Hard surfaces should be avoided. Successful jogging depends on fitness, age and endurance. Study the subject carefully, and jog under the auspices of your local Sports Centre if you have one.

Golf

Golf is a good fresh air activity which mobilises the body and hips and increases flexibility and co-ordination. It is a fairly mild form of exercise, unless the course is hilly or you are competitive. However, it can help to release tension.

Tennis

Tennis is good for heart and lungs as a keen player has to run about a great deal. Here again, the not-so-young need to watch foot, ankle and leg muscles as tendons and ligaments cannot take too much pounding. And watch that tennis elbow. Any injuries, however minor, should be treated at once.

Walking

Sometimes I think that walking beats all the other open air types of exercise. You don't need special clothes, only flat-heeled shoes, a raincoat and a scarf and you are away. You are independent of any machine, partner, racquet, club or cancelled arrangement. You are free to go at any time, anywhere you wish. If you walk briskly from the hips, consciously stepping it out with your head up and your arms uncluttered and swinging, it's wonderful. You are working at least fifty percent of your muscles, and making your lungs work harder. You can set your own pace, and to my mind you can't beat it. It improves your looks too!

Cycling

If you happen to be a keen cyclist, then you have a lot going for you, and you are certainly strengthening your leg muscles as well as being able to go to places out of reach for the walker. Cycling, like walking, jogging, swimming, and similar activities, strengthens the lungs and heart by making them work harder. However, before attempting a really long ride, or before buying a bicycle for the first time, my advice is to limber up with the exercises in Chapter 14. You will need all your stamina and strength.

Warning

If you start gently and don't overdo it, my exercises will not cause any problems, but if you take up a new sport and go all out from the start, you will get a little muscle soreness. It takes time to get back into condition. Don't give up or proceed in spite of feeling sore. Just take things a little more easily.

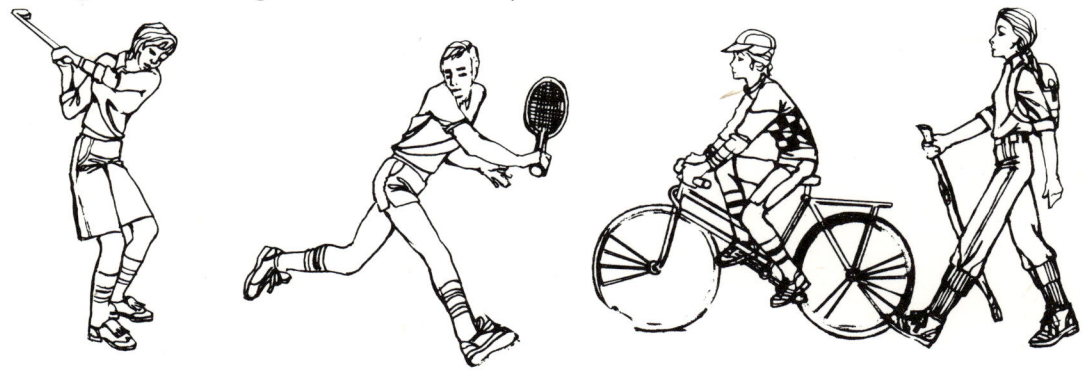

Correct breathing

Exercise is closely linked with breathing, and deep breaths of fresh air are essential for good health.

At one time when exercising we would raise our arms up sideways while breathing in and lower them while breathing out, but the entire structure of modern exercises and movement has changed and become more fluid, and we no longer talk about 'breathing' as such. When we move in this more relaxed manner, we just let the breathing happen. We breathe naturally. Exercises with a moving base such as skipping, running, hopping or dancing can get you a little out of breath, but this is good for you provided you do not allow yourself to become exhausted.

Breathing practice has now become something very special and many people follow the yoga pattern and make it part of their daily lives. Quite apart from the fact that deep and controlled breathing is essential to health, it has a tremendously relaxing effect. There has been many a time before a countdown in front of television cameras when I have been grateful for the habit of deep breathing. It has a very calming effect on the nerves.

It is important to remember that shallow breathing is dangerous as the lungs are never fully used, and the residue of used-up air is always there. Learn to breathe deeply. Instead of inhaling first, start by exhaling fully. Breathe out as you would if you were collapsing a balloon. When you feel that your lungs are entirely empty, breathe in deeply and steadily, and go on breathing in until you feel that your lungs will burst. Hold your breath while you count three, then let it go completely and start all over again. Deep breathing exercises are intended for those people whose breathing capacity is normal. If any dizziness or shortage of breath is experienced when doing the exercise, it would be wise to seek a doctor's advice.

Try to breathe in really fresh air and then the oxygen content will be greater and will facilitate the elimination of waste products. Always breathe through the nose so that the nasal passages can do their job of trapping the millions of particles of dust and dirt; breathing through the mouth can lead to congested sinuses, sore throats and other infections.

Deep breathing can help you to sleep if you are wakeful at night. I have known six really complete breaths succeed when all other methods have failed.

Incidentally, deep breathing followed by a couple of favourite exercises, or changing to a practical job, can clear your head if you are suffering from mental fatigue. Body rest is not the answer – you need a fresh supply of blood and oxygen, and that means exercise.

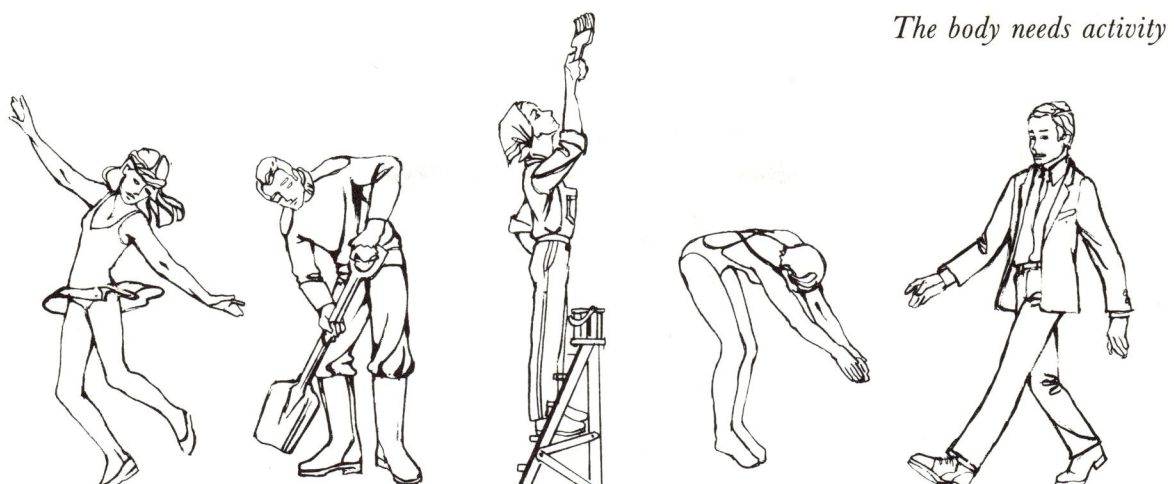

Active leisure

The more I see of families who make a hobby out of exercise and active leisure, the more impressed I am with their youthful looks and vigour. They have that special something that others don't always have – a lift of the head, a ready smile, a confident walk. Their attitude to life is more positive; they will work during the years when most people retire; they are busy giving their services; they know that movement is life and that the body needs activity.

I am not sure that active leisure isn't a better term than exercise when applied to the family. Many women have a natural feeling for moving to music, but men usually prefer an objective when they use their muscles. Children tend to follow suit; the daughter goes to a dancing class and the boy plays football. But they are all moving, keeping themselves fit and agile, and at the same time counteracting the ill effects of too much sitting. Little girls (and boys) who start to dance at an early age are lucky: they develop poise and confidence and are much less likely to be gauche, shy or just plain clumsy later on.

Facilities for swimming (an essential skill for an island race, I believe), athletics and sports are getting better all the time. If a Sports Centre is within reach, it is well worth the whole family taking advantage of what it has to offer. (See Chapter 19.)

Local keep fit classes make splendid outlets for women. There is usually a very strong social atmosphere at these classes, for all age groups, and plenty of opportunities to visit other groups, attend rallies, arrange parties and generally have an enjoyable time. The keep fit plan inevitably spreads to the rest of the family. 'Show us what you do, Mum,' and in many homes furniture is pushed back, on goes a popular record or tape and everyone joins in. Even the masculine element will say, 'No, that's kids' stuff,' and show you what they can do. The exercises for strength, mobility and good posture are suitable for everyone.

There are always the day to day activities, such as walking, gardening, cleaning the car or taking the dog out, which are very valuable as a form of life insurance and should be kept up long after the children have left home. Men enjoy vigorous sports and are often responsible for gardening and cleaning the car. If you have an aptitude for painting or carpentry, for example, this can be an excellent 'active' leisure occupation if it makes you stretch or bend your knees!

The right food

Eating the right food means eating sensibly to suit one's needs. It is true that one man's meat is another man's poison, and who is to say what is right for each particular stomach. It always amazes me how one person can enjoy a meal that would put someone else in bed for a week! Thousands of people's lives are haunted by the effort to diet, and even more incredibly by the need to buy tablets for indigestion. Many people carry them around, just in case.

To many, sensible eating is worth a ransom. It is a way to be fitter and slimmer at the same time, to present a new image to those we care about and to improve our approach to life. It gives us an interest in the way we dress, and it makes us feel younger, smarter and less tired. To others, let's face it, sensible eating is a discipline, a giving up of what some people say is their main joy in life; all the lovely food and drink that they once considered a luxury they now cannot do without.

Eating for health can be so rewarding; you feel well, you have no indigestion, no swelling stomach, no extra pounds in weight. Your skin and eyes are clear, and you have a wonderful feeling of get up and go. Give me the lighter meals, the natural things – eggs, fish, cheese, fruit, vegetables, yoghurt, brown bread. There is an enormous variety of delicious sensible foods that will, when combined with exercise, ensure a firm chin line, non-sagging upper arms, slim ankles and a flat tummy. I include an excellent high-fibre diet in Chapter 4, which concentrates on these natural healthy foods.

It is quite possible to eat a great deal of food and yet be deficient in the vitamins, minerals, proteins and roughage that the body needs. Many people with large appetites, for both food and drink, look very healthy but are the first to suffer from diseases of the heart. They may take in tremendous amounts of vitamins, but the rest of their diet is not a balanced one.

Food fanatics may be dull, but it is not fanatical to eat wisely and well. Circulatory problems are often put down to eating too much animal fat. Too much refined sugar is linked with cholesterol build-up. Too many junk and starchy foods should be avoided, but a completely vegetarian diet can bring problems of insufficient protein during later life.

Relaxation

Oh, the joy of it, to be able to relax at will. What a gift! How lucky are those people who, at the height of their tension, stop talking, close their eyes and let go. Is it only a gift? Well, the good news is that relaxation can be learnt. To master tension has never been easy, but, strangely enough, it can be done through exercise. This may sound like a paradox, but it is not.

Learning how to relax properly is a fundamental part of keeping fit. First, you have to recognise the meaning of tension; to know when your shoulders are up instead of down; to realise that the back of your neck is beginning to feel stiff and to hurt, that your hands are not still, and that you are shifting about in your chair because your lower back is giving you trouble. All these miseries come from feeling tense. The tossing and turning in bed and the inability to sleep can be caused by worry over problems that cannot be solved. Tension takes over and one seems powerless to do anything about it. But you can, if you try. If you are willing to practise, you can learn to let go – little by little, muscle by muscle – until a welcome lethargy takes over and you can rest.

Perhaps the hardest part of this training is to prevent the mind from wandering. I find it essential to concentrate on each group of muscles, one by one, but methods of relaxing differ according to the individual's needs. Some people prefer to lie very still and repeat a word or phrase; others think about beautiful scenes, mountains, the sea, gentle breezes or the humming of bees. These thoughts can be very relaxing, but if they arouse memories, pleasant or otherwise, they can stimulate the brain, and this stimulation should be avoided at all costs. Once the brain begins to work it goes on working, and tension builds up again. Very tense people find that their muscles are tight even when they sleep. They sleep with their hands clenched, heads dug into pillows and backs stiff; waking is a painful business. The mental exhaustion which comes from being tense is easy to understand when you consider how close to each other are the mind and body. Because of this, tension cannot fail to have an effect on the nerves.

Relaxation
Lie on the floor with
both feet up on the seat
of an armchair or
cushioned stool.

Yet, when we learn to relax we can 'let go' physically and stop worrying, and feel at peace with the world.

Have you ever tried rubbing the nape of your neck very gently, smoothing your fingers over the nerve centres at the base of your skull? It always makes me yawn. Lying on the floor with your feet up is relaxing. And the hand movements in Chapter 7 help when hands are tense: make a fist, stretch your fingers and then shake them gently from the wrist.

These are the little tricks, but we need a number of tricks to allay tension. Will-power alone is not the answer. You cannot force a muscle to relax, you have to train it to do so. So we are back to exercise. We have to feel for ourselves when tension is present and when relaxation takes its place. Try it now.

Take a deep breath and tense up all the muscles in your body. Hold the position for several seconds – feel the tension – feel your muscles tightening up – imagine a terrible catastrophe – feel frightened – and then exhale. Let your breath go with a long sigh and *feel* the tension seeping out of your muscles. *Feel* the difference. This is the first step. The imagined danger is past, so sit comfortably or lie flat on your back.

Another way to recognise tension is to hold out your arm stiffly at shoulder height and go on holding it there for several seconds, unsupported. Then let the arm drop and feel the utter relief.

Now for the training. Tell your feet to go to sleep. Say, out loud if you are alone, 'Go to sleep feet, you are so heavy that I cannot lift you.' Move on and upwards covering knees, back, shoulders, arms, until you reach your head. Heads are very heavy and it is important to feel that your head is made of lead. Now feel that you are falling, falling through the floor. Talk yourself into a completely relaxed state. Practise at every opportunity and you will master the skill.

Sound sleep

It is difficult to separate relaxation from sound sleep, as one follows the other. You cannot sleep unless you are relaxed. However, you can do several things to ensure a good night's rest apart from learning the technique of relaxation. Just as with the choice of foods, people's requirements vary. Some cannot close their eyes without the burden of heavy bed clothes, a warm room and windows closely curtained. Others would lie awake all night unless coverings were warm but very light, the window open and curtains drawn back. But what of those who have tried everything – socks, hot water bottles, reading until all hours, late-night radio music, going to bed at dusk and getting up at dawn? Insomnia is a very serious problem because exercise, fresh air and sensible eating are of no avail if you cannot get a good night's sound sleep. But you can, if you learn to relax.

Fatigue is a poison and a killer, and unless you are very young it shows in the unkindest ways possible: a colourless skin, rings round the eyes and a tendency to slump round the middle; then the shoulders sag, the bust gets nearer to the waist, and behold, the unsightly roll which precedes a thickening of the figure. Fatigue is the enemy of beauty and it usually attacks when we insist on going on too long – the late-night television programme, that last row of knitting, the book that should be put down. If this stage of tiredness is reached, there is only one answer. Rest – or the tiredness will persist and build into chronic fatigue.

So how do you get more rest? The first essential is to learn how to relax, so follow my suggestions and practise this relaxation technique whenever you feel overtired and tense. Study your bedroom, window space, ventilation, heating, lighting – anything that is the slightest aggravation. Are the curtains right, or do they let in too much light, or too little? Does it worry you if the window is open or closed? Do the boards creak? How is the plumbing? Does someone else keep you awake? No detail is too small when it comes to sleeping. We will never be really fit if we cannot sleep.

To my mind, the popularity of the duvet has helped very many people to sleep better. Being tucked in heavy bedclothes can give you cramp, and a bad back if you are not careful how you turn. If you throw off the bedclothes you are liable to catch a cold. A duvet is warm, light and very practical. Sleep was my problem until my keep-fit friends persuaded me to give up my electric blanket and buy a duvet – and I have slept well ever since.

Another aid to sound sleep is a warm milky drink. It is also very important to allow yourself sufficient time to go to bed gradually. It is the slowing down process that is so helpful, the routine of preparation. Make time to look after yourself, to scrupulously cleanse the skin and the teeth, to brush the hair, to gently massage and cream the face and neck. All these things take a little time and they slow you down and help to quieten any tension. The time spent is made up by getting to sleep more quickly, and looking better in the morning.

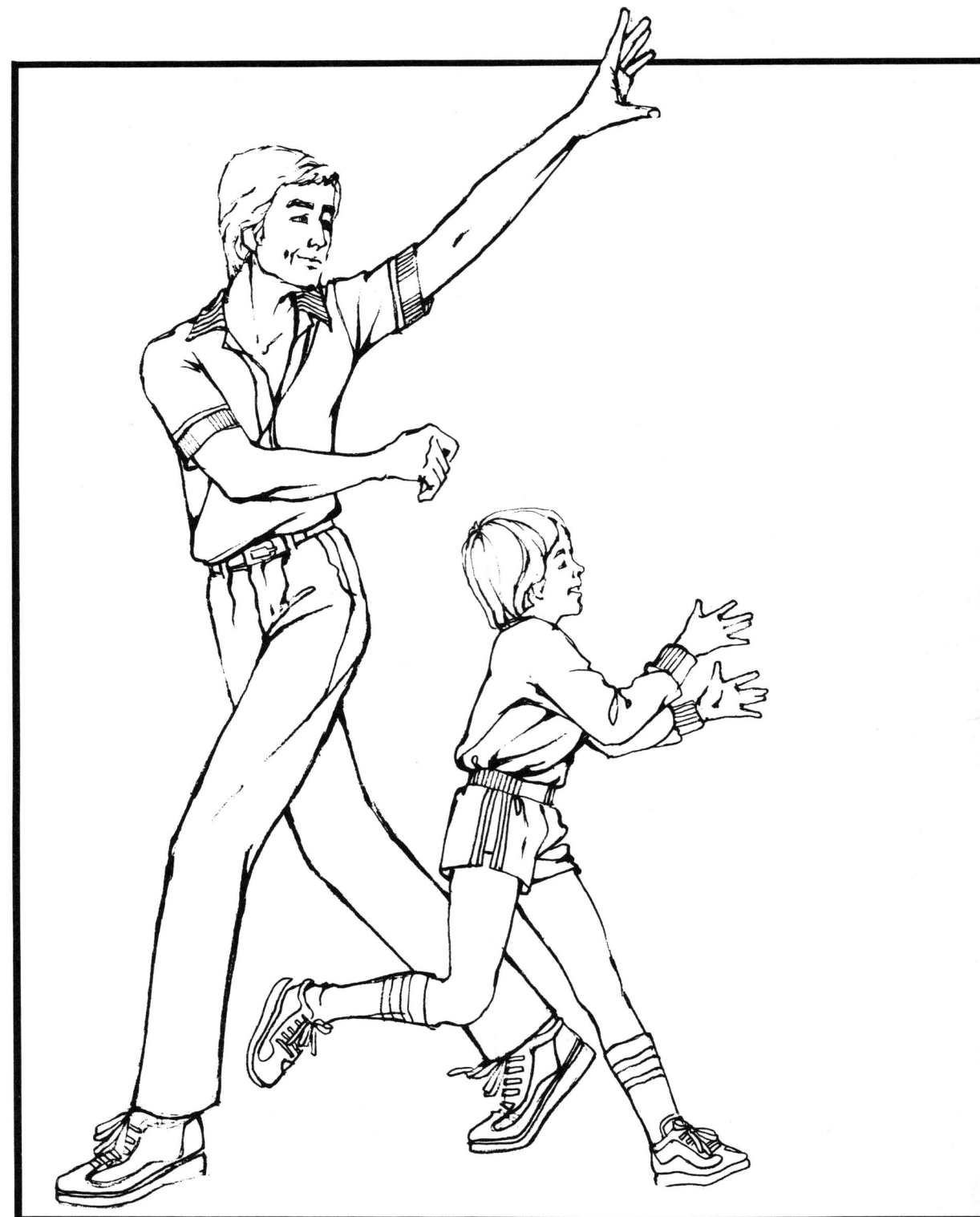

Chapter 2

Family fitness

Encourage children to be active. Overweight children make overweight adults. Adolescence and poor posture. Women and exercise. Men's need for health, strength and stamina. Exercise and the older generation.

Most children today are healthy animals who kick a ball about, cycle, swim, run, jump and generally keep themselves fit. Then comes adolescence, and with it a period of very fast growth. Those who are tall often develop a tendency to stoop and become round-shouldered. You have to have confidence to stand tall, and many boys and girls in their early teens are very self-conscious. In Victorian times, with a book on the head or a board at the back, discipline took care of good posture, stiff and starchy though it was. Nowadays, if parents are keen on outdoor activities, some of their enthusiasm will brush off on their children and they will learn to accept the value of exercise rather than laugh at the idea.

Most bad habits, such as standing badly and overeating develop early and are difficult to eradicate. It can be tiresome and boring continually to correct a disinterested child, but it is well worth the trouble. I have always found that if you continue to instil the golden rules for long enough, some of them eventually take root! It is much the same with fitness. If you encourage a child to join in all kinds of activities, such as sport, swimming, games or camping, he or she will always find something that they like to do. A love of the open air and an urge for active pastimes can be fostered at a very early age.

Independence

A certain amount of independence is a good thing for everyone, and learning to be responsible in small ways is a wonderful training for what will be needed later on in life. In an increasingly competitive world we simply cannot rely on other people. I feel that every boy and girl today should be equipped for a very special tomorrow and have modern skills and resources within himself. He should want to work and be excited about his future. He should have time for exercise and a healthy way of life, and he should be able to look after himself so that, whatever transpires, he will be independent.

Fit not fat

There are some highly intelligent children who will choose to study while others are playing games. Provided that their metabolic rates are high and they use up naturally food that other children have to work off, then overweight should never be a problem. The problems arise when a child is bursting out of his clothes but at the same time tends to be lazy. Due to such factors as television, cars, lifts and escalators etc, there has been a big drop in activity levels over the last decade and it has been said that there are more overweight youngsters today than there have been at any time in the past. And it has been proved that many overweight children become overweight men and women.

I frequently join a panel of judges to choose the Golden Slimmer of the Year. Usually eight finalists compete for the annual award. We, the judges, interrogate them as to why and how they have been able to lose eight, nine or ten stones and shed their horrific fat. Time and again, men and women will tell you their problem started in childhood when they were told to 'Eat up, dear, you'll never be a big boy/girl if you don't,' and sure enough, they ate and became big.

They tell you that they needed an incentive to start slimming. One lovely finalist told me that all the little boys in her son's class at school were making aprons as Christmas presents for their mothers. When he produced his own mother's measurements there wasn't enough material left to make it. He came home crying – she dried his tears and then decided to slim.

I have always believed that the key to a child's future good health comes from within the family. Encourage children to enjoy simple wholesome food and cut down on those foods that are not good for them. Try to eliminate from their diet the fried foods, gooey cakes, sweets and packaged goods with all their preservatives. If children are offered fruit and vegetables, grilled fish, lean meat, milk and eggs early enough, they will accept them, enjoy them and grow up expecting to eat that way. Many children prefer plain food anyway, and low-calorie savoury dishes can be just as exciting to them as more fatty and starchy meals.

Children will usually choose to eat good healthy foods rather than be ridiculed for being overweight. You get the occasional fat boy or girl destined to be the life and soul of the party, but most children are very sensitive about their appearance and hate to be different from the others. If they are too heavy, they are probably lackadaisical and wild horses would not drag them out to exercise or to play energetic games. But they might change their eating habits if they realised that it meant being one of the (active) crowd. A child needs to be accepted by the group, to be neither out in front nor completely in the background. Once the extra pounds have gone, the energy will be there, and with it the will to have a go and the desire to join in. The slimmer child will be fitter and happier in every way.

Adolescence

In adolescence the picture changes; life becomes either very exciting or quite unbearable. Gymnastics and games become less attractive, possibly because games are a bit too competitive, and no goals are scored or awards won. Boys yearn for motorbikes and girls reach for lipstick. Actually, these new interests are a good sign; many a girl keeps fit for the sake of her appearance, and the male is not alone in his desire to show off a manly chest and mighty muscles. Energy is channelled into creative, not competitive, activity. To keep fit and on the move at home, Chapter 13, 'Dance mobility', includes three exhilarating routines based on disco and pop music.

Posture problems

Suddenly, a boy's height matters. Maybe the girlfriend is tall, and he has to look up to her, and even if it is a case of 'eyes level' he will still wish that it were not so. It may not have occurred to him that he might be slightly round-shouldered and could gain height by standing straighter. Good posture is a must, and so are exercises to strengthen the supporting muscles. Chapters 9 and 14 contain some useful movements for improving posture and making the most of one's height. The chosen exercises should be practised daily.

Today's willowy teenage girls have a greater problem because they have to counteract a tendency to stoop. Many tall girls have 'model' measurements and ambitions in this direction. But whatever the calling, it is imperative to stand tall or ruin a lovely figure. I would advise starting with the Shoulder Test in Chapter 1. Follow this with the Climbing Claps: stretch upwards with both arms and clap overhead three times, getting higher and higher, and feel the bust pulling up and away from the hips – then let the arms come down sideways. Repeat several times at any odd moment.

Rolling the shoulders back in circles, and circling the arm backwards one at a time will correct any tendency to stoop. Do these exercises several times a day to ensure an excellent upright stance.

Heavy bags slung over one shoulder can lead to a one-sided position which destroys good posture. Even school books can be heavy and make it easy to slouch. Uneven weight distribution over a long period can become ugly and painful and set up all kinds of strain and stress in years to come. Think of campers and walkers who are much more comfortable carrying their load high

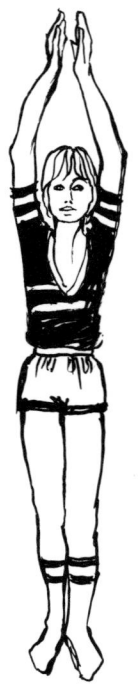

Climbing claps
Raise both arms up sideways. Reach up and clap 3 times overhead, getting higher and higher. Arms down and repeat.

on their backs, with two straps – just as some Eastern women (and some Western) carry their babies!

Although young backs are usually strong backs, full development is still taking place and great care should be taken when carrying heavy bags or picking up heavy objects from ground level. Bending forward puts great strain upon the area around the base of the spine. Muscles and ligaments can be overstretched, setting up painful inflammation. The knees must be bent, and the object to be lifted should be held close to the body for extra support. In this way the legs take some of the strain.

Fitness for adults

Some men and women move well naturally, but not all; good movement is a skill which is well worth learning. Clumsy, erratic and tense ways of going about a job help neither the job nor you, and in many cases lead to accidents which might have been prevented. Too many accidents happen in the home, and this is one reason why I believe in a daily exercise routine. Out-of-door activities help us to keep healthy, but learning to control our body movements is something else.

My exercises will extend your range of movement so that reaching for something high up or low down will be easy. They will improve your balance and recovery should you slip; they will help you to mobilise the upper back and shoulders (when, say, a period of ironing or working over a bench leaves the muscles in spasm and momentarily very painful); hands and fingers will loosen up and strengthen with the little exercises; backs will benefit when hips, legs and feet are under your control. You can stand at ease. Tension will be less and there will never be an ugly or poky movement.

In addition to the benefits the different parts of your body will experience, you will also look good while you are moving or standing because you will have taken your new-found knowledge into your daily life. Your posture will improve automatically, and you will have a spring in your step, more energy and more vitality.

Women

Most women hate household chores, but if you think of them as a means of improving your appearance and mobility, they are not half as bad! So stay active – don't be an onlooker. Sitting around and looking pretty won't mean a thing later on. Actually, it's highly dangerous because inactivity can become a habit, and many a slim young girl has had to fight overweight later in life. Generally speaking, don't despise the chores, despise the armchairs. Having said this, I must make it clear that I am not in favour of strenuous exercise for women at all times. It doesn't suit everyone. But as I have said before, our modern method is beneficial because it is strengthening without being exhausting.

Whenever I have been asked by a woman whether she should attend Keep Fit classes or exercise during her period, I do not say 'Yes' out of hand. If you are in pain or feel utterly drained, rest is the answer. However – and I mean this – if you are suffering from pre-menstrual tension, exercising to music works wonders.

I have also been asked whether really fit women suffer fewer miscarriages and have shorter labour. One cannot possibly generalise and I am of the opinion that this is a medical issue, but I am convinced that being unfit will not help. In cases of pregnancy, many mothers have told me how much they have been helped by their keep fit exercises.

A doctor or local Health Authority will give specific advice regarding exercises during pregnancy. They are taught, preferably after the third month, in the physiotherapy department of some hospitals, at health centres, local clinics, or by a midwife or health visitor. Certainly no pregnant women should do exercises without medical advice if she has a history of miscarriage or threatened abortion. As your exercises will affect certain muscles, it is important to get proper advice and to take every precaution when expecting a child.

Post-natal exercises are taught by staff at maternity hospitals, usually after the first 24 hours if the birth is normal. Full exercise or exertion should not be undertaken until after the final post-natal examination at six weeks. Mothers can usually return to their regular keep fit routines within three to six months. If starting to exercise earlier, I would suggest starting with the relaxing routine in Chapter 17, the chair exercises in Chapter 18 and Morning Choice (Chapter 16). Care must be taken to avoid over-stretching or too vigorous abdominal exercise. Aim for good posture.

Why should men exercise?

Men should exercise because they need to be fit – and don't we all? More often than not, however, the man is the main breadwinner in the family, and his health, strength and endurance are vital to his life and work. He needs the support of an active and healthy body. Exercise increases physical endurance and stamina and also gives greater reserves of energy for enjoying leisure pursuits.

Areas which need attention are the muscles of shoulders, arms, abdomen, back and legs, and the heart, lungs and blood vessels. A simple fitness scheme suitable for most men would be active participation in one or two sports, supplemented by a balanced set of exercises. Limbering up for different sports can stretch and strengthen the muscles. If sport is not a possibility, it becomes essential to spare a few minutes each day to keep active and in good condition. To my mind, many men age too soon; exercise will keep them young.

These days, many men are more involved with the progress and well-being of their children than they were in the past. They no longer feel that it is undignified to be seen pushing a perambulator or reining in a tiny tot. Young men interested in sport and outdoor activities make splendid fathers because they like to take their children along and are quite prepared to share their games and encourage them to be as active as possible.

Grandparents

The importance of exercise for the older generation is covered fully in Chapter 7.

In the context of the family, the grandparents very often influence the children when it comes to exercise and keeping fit. Most know and accept the value of an active life and will teach the rudiments of cricket or football with all the patience in the world. Less helpful are those who take to the armchair in middle life, and instead of making an effort to play with the youngsters they say, 'You run along, I've got a bone in my leg.' Children are mimics and learn what is what very early. If we don't join in, they will associate us with age and put us right on top of the shelf.

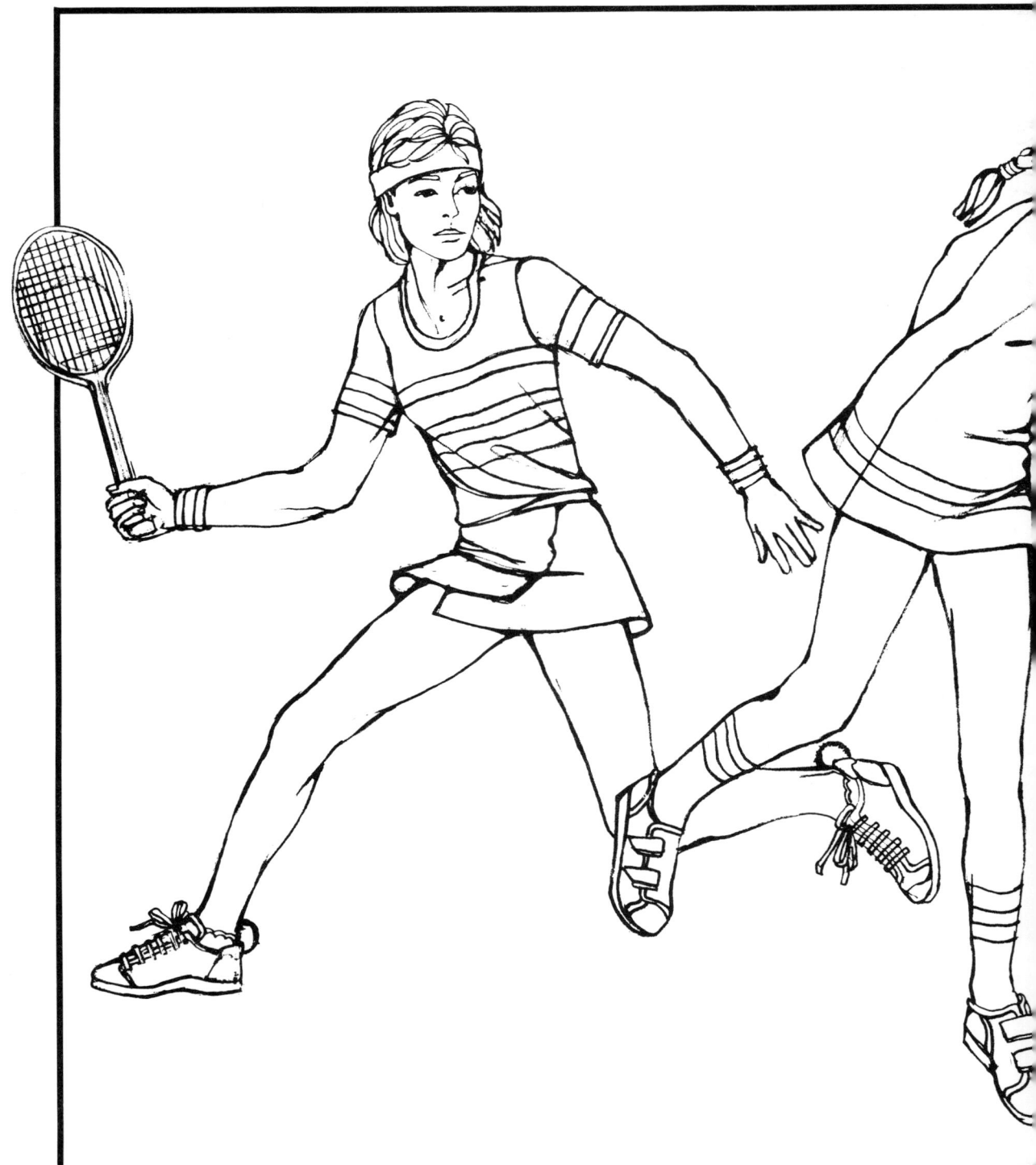

Chapter 3

Keeping fit
as a way of life

**Keeping fit keeps you young. The 'think
young and stay young' philosophy. The
benefits of being fit.
Do not take good health for granted.
Exercise to strengthen heart and lungs and
to bring a feeling of exhilaration.
Use exercise as an antidote to mental
fatigue. Exercise to eliminate aches and
pains brought on by tension.
Fill your lungs with fresh air,
avoid cigarette smoke.**

Perhaps the most outstanding benefit to be gained from a keep fit way of life is that it keeps you young. From this, all other benefits spring. The preoccupation with age today is widespread. The years are carefully counted, and many lives are limited because of an old-fashioned conception of age. Why? It no longer follows that because you are forty, fifty, sixty or seventy you cannot be young in mind, spirit and body. Of course you can. The bounds are not set. We have grown up with these fallacies and preconceived ideas, and have been brain-washed regarding the ageing processes. If we think that we are bound to deteriorate day by day, then we will. Nothing can stop us getting old because we are controlled by our thoughts. It is our outlook that counts; the way we think and our attitude towards life that is so important. Think young and stay young is my philosophy.

Men and women are often so age-conscious that the worry and fear of the future shows in their faces. Those people who become very tense about ageing will even shop for the kind of clothes they think they ought to wear, not the ones they really want. They are afraid to alter their appearance because they feel that a modern look is too young for them. Getting set in one's ideas and resting in a rut is tantamount to saying, 'I'm getting on, you know.'

Fortunately, you don't find this state of affairs in the keep fit world. Getting into a leotard or stylish pair of trousers for a keep fit class makes women more figure-conscious, so that if you are overweight you do something about it! You learn to move in a more youthful way, so you begin to look younger. Maybe some of your clothes feel a bit old-fashioned, so you go for something more up-to-date. The group leader wants you to take part in a demonstration, so you try a new hair style – and hey presto! You look and feel years younger. You watch what you eat, jig around at home to music on the radio, and you look at your contemporaries and say, 'Did I really look like that?'

The same goes for men too. Those who are keen on fitness, fresh air and activity usually move with the times. They delight everyone with their younger and more casual appearance. Somehow the years drop away and are forgotten. Staying young is really maintenance, and you cannot start too soon.

Maintenance

Mercifully, when you are young you don't think about age, except to grow up as quickly as possible. Energy, vitality and a youthful appearance are the young person's natural assets, and you cannot imagine ever looking old. Well, you will not look old if you make it your business, or hobby, to keep what you have got. Use your vitality and energy to keep your muscles as well toned-up in the future as they are today.

Maintenance is a must. Whether it is your house, your car, your dog or yourself, it has to be maintained or the costs will be high. Everything costs more to put right if it has been neglected, and most of all ourselves. If we let the roof go, there's a big bill to pay when we eventually send for the builder, but replace a slate and the cost is minimal. All my life I have found maintenance to be the operative word. 'Stop the rot' has been my motto. Another which has always been important to me is, 'Do it now'. I have talked to many doctors on the subject of health maintenance and prevention of illness and all say without question, 'Tell us about it now, not in six months' time.'

Good circulation

Exercise strengthens the heart and lungs. It peps up the circulation, makes one breathe more deeply, and brings with it a feeling of exhilaration. Hair and skin improve too.

To keep our minds working at top speed the brain benefits from anything we do that ensures a good supply of blood and oxygen. Without this, it cannot function efficiently. Good circulation, essential for good health, becomes more and more important as the years go by, and is a very good reason why we should keep moving and keep exercising. If you are fit at fifty and you are prepared to keep active then there is every chance that, barring accidents or disease, you should be just as fit at seventy or eighty. Overweight and lack of fitness can put a strain on the heart and can result in high blood pressure and all the related problems.

Concentration

Fitness first also means safety first. Even if you are not keen on exercises, don't forget that they train concentration and balance and keep you alert. Exercises train the muscles that will hold you still, suddenly, at a dangerous road crossing; they will give you mobile feet that will carry you safely in front of a fast-moving vehicle, or root you to the spot in an emergency. Oh yes, keep fit has many facets. It's worth learning the skill.

Anticipation

You have to anticipate, check and do something *before* it happens. Some people don't have their cars checked often enough; I try to renew my brakes before they go, not afterwards. It's too late when you can't stop. Anticipation works with everything. If you want to be fit and you want to stay young, don't wait until you are sick or getting old before doing something about it. Anticipate and prevent it happening. Keep yourself looking good and feeling good – it's ugly to let yourself go. It's the same with your problems: don't sew up your life because you cannot see where you are going. Think, plan, check, anticipate.

Fitness for success

Everybody wants to be successful at something. Whether your ambition is for international stardom, to grow the largest marrow, or to help finance the aged, the message is much the same. You will need courage, determination and patience. In addition, you will need to be very fit; you will need stamina, both physical and mental.

Never take your good health for granted, but value it above rubies. Good health will keep you feeling good and looking good all the time, and it is one of life's basic needs.

I have seen many people achieve success, and they have nearly always been strong and sturdy. They have had to be strong enough to stand the strain of jetting halfway across the world, coping with a variety of climates, long days and short nights. They were not always the most talented or beautiful, but they knew how to take care of themselves. They had prepared for success, and taken the trouble to follow the rules. They were fit. They made time in their busy lives for plenty of exercise and fresh air. They carried nothing to excess and as far as possible they ate the right food, and learnt to relax – they had to. Great occasions and long work sessions found them fit and ready – and, above all, confident.

Communication

Another route to success is communication. The friendly approach is invaluable; the art of communication is priceless. A bold statement, maybe, but how many appalling situations have been saved by someone who can reach you; someone not necessarily on your side but someone who is so warm and friendly that you are convinced that they really care. So you listen. What a gift this is.

I know a person who meets you and greets you as if all day she has been waiting to do just that. Her warm light-hearted 'Hallo' gives everyone a lift. She smiles and laughs, forgetful of any problems she may have, only interested in you. She is not waiting for you to stop talking with growing impatience, anxious to get a word in, wrapped up in herself. She is communicating, giving her time to you. It is no effort; she is fitness itself. Her love of fresh air, exercise, swimming and dancing has been shared with her family and her two sons. Some would say, 'She is a natural,' and they would be right. But I know hundreds more (I could truthfully say thousands), who have come to terms with the six essentials – exercise, fresh air, active leisure, the right food, relaxation and sound sleep – and have the same friendly approach, the same light in their eyes, and the same desire to communicate.

Confidence

Fitness brings with it poise and confidence. It gives you vitality. It makes you look good and it adds a spring to the step. If you are confident then friendships become easier and shyness and loneliness can be overcome.

Man or woman, adolescent or pensioner, life is easier if you are a good mixer. I have talked to so many people who are surprisingly shy. They are all charming people who find it difficult to be at ease with strangers and find it impossible to go halfway to meet them. The shy ones want to join in, and would love to ask you to their homes, but somehow they don't. If they go to a party, they listen to every word that is spoken, but are never quick enough to get one in themselves. Reams have been written about gaining a confident approach, but there is an invisible wall which prevents them from taking advantage of all this advice. Invite

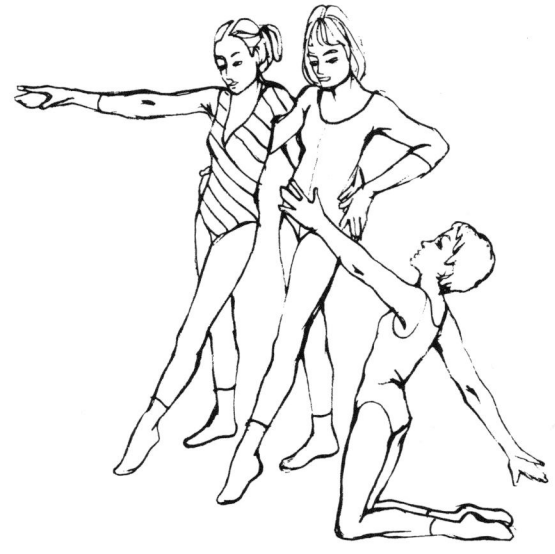

Keep fit classes
Keep fit classes exist in most towns and villages. Women of all ages are welcome.

such a person to a keep fit class and she'll say, 'Oh no, I couldn't go there,' or 'I wouldn't like to wear a leotard.'

These are the shy ones, the nice ones who are missing out on us – and we are missing out on them. They are usually modest, and modesty pays. How long can you bear the stand-up comic, the shouter, the boaster, the life and soul of the party? It is far more exciting to find out gradually about someone's achievements than to have them told to you on first meeting. But it is inevitable, if the shyness stays, that he or she will have periods of great loneliness.

You have guessed my remedy. Join a club, a keep fit class, a Sports Centre, anything that is outgoing. When you are moving to music or kicking a ball, shyness doesn't come into it. You are too busy to worry. You are part of something positive and alive. You have made an effort to mix and you are building a more vital, attractive and welcoming personality.

Tension relief

We all suffer from mental fatigue from time to time and deep breathing followed by a few exercises is an excellent antidote. The fresh supply of blood and oxygen to heart and lungs will do more good than any alcoholic drink or comfortable armchair. Recognise the tension and develop a relaxation routine and make it part of your daily life.

If you have a sedentary job, use exercise to eliminate the little aches and pains brought on by tension. Neck and shoulders stiffen if kept in one position for too long; they hurt if you have to twist the same way to read when typing, and ache if your head is constantly bent over your work. Heads are terribly heavy and the supporting neck muscles will ache if asked to hold this weight in any position other than the correct one. These pains should be dealt with as soon as they are felt; they will only get worse as tension builds.

The best treatment for aching neck and shoulders is to take a few minutes off and move. If you can, stand up and stretch, swing or walk about then instant relief will be felt; if not, do some of my chair exercises (see Chapter 18).

Another excellent exercise is to turn your head gently from side to side, and look all round the room – high up and in every direction. Shrug your shoulders up and down and roll them backwards in little circles. Make that upper back so mobile that it cannot get set and give pain. Keep moving. At the same time, make sure that your back is supported at the base of the spine. Back problems of the future will be influenced by the way you are sitting now.

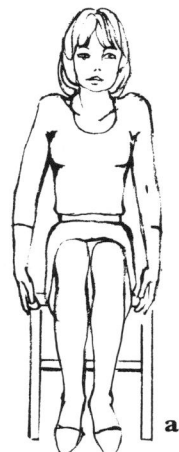 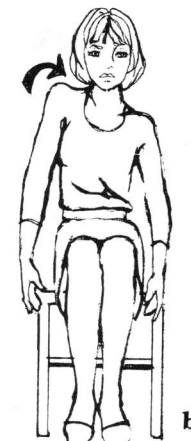 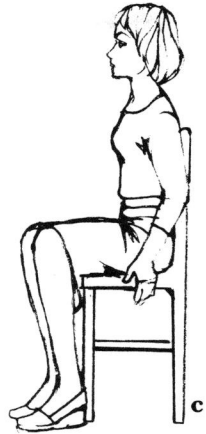

a Shrug your shoulders up to your ears and down.
b Lift each shoulder, roll back and round in circles.
c Sit with base of spine supported by back of chair.

Smoking

Many people say that smoking helps them relax. It is estimated that up to 30,000 cases of lung cancer *caused by smoking* are registered in Britain every year, and you know the usual result. Of these, many sufferers don't even reach retirement age let alone live a long life. Bronchitis is another killer, and so are emphysema, chest illnesses and weakened hearts. All these dreadful illnesses can be caused because we think that smoking soothes our nerves. What a price to pay for a bit of relaxation. Pregnant women damage their babies; it repels rather than attracts; it is a horrible habit. You cannot smoke and be truly fit. Have you ever seen anyone gasp for breath, unable to get air into lifeless lungs?

Please, please keep your lungs healthy. Fill them with fresh air not cigarette smoke. It is so easy to say 'Stop smoking!' but so difficult for those to give up who want to. Most people wait until they have to – and it is often too late.

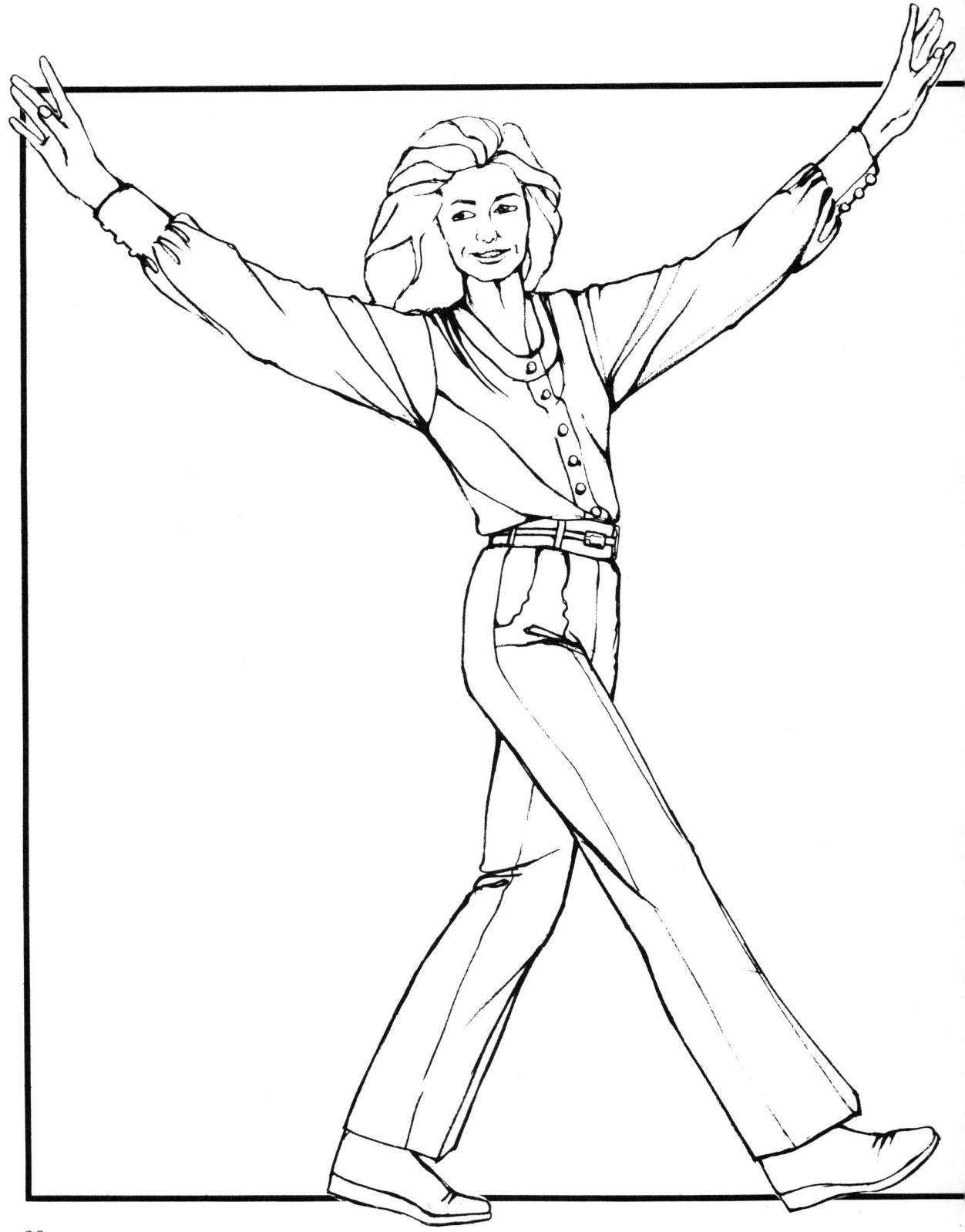

Chapter 4

Be fit, slim and happy

To promote energy you must be fit; to conserve it you must be fit. Turn fitness to your advantage. Let energy give you confidence. Fight against depression. Tackle the gloom and let in some light.
Play truant. Everyone needs a change.
The problems and dangers of overweight.
Bodies get even.
Keep fit foods and a high fibre diet.
Eating for health and figure is only half the story – exercise is the other half.

I f you are fit and used to being energetic you can use this to your advantage. You can always do something if things become difficult, even in cases of redundancy. The more energy you have, the less likely you are to feel depressed or unwanted. Energy gives you confidence; you don't want to sit around, you want to be up and doing, learning a new skill, doing up the house, overhauling the car, growing vegetables, a thousand things.

The fitness requirements of men and women are much the same. To promote energy, we must be fit; to conserve it, we must be fit. We need to aim for strength, flexibility, endurance, mobility, co-ordination and weight control. We need a knowledge of nutrition and a capacity for relaxation, and out of this will come the energy to do what we want to do and what we have to do.

Depression

Why is it that some people never seem to be depressed? They will moan in a humorous kind of way about their various problems but will finish up with a rueful smile, 'Oh well,' they will say, 'everything passes,' and it does. They are the survivors, the people who refuse to be got down. They know that the good, the bad and the indifferent will eventually pass. It is not much comfort at the time, but how often have we looked back and wondered how we managed to get through? Somehow we survived, but it's not always easy to remember this, and at times we get depressed. Perhaps nothing is terribly wrong, but nothing seems terribly right. It is usually the little things that become so important on not-so-good days: someone has not telephoned; that chap at work has been insensitive; the state of your hair depresses you. Birthdays upset some people – another year gone! If you are feeling very low, you actually *look* for the extra lines on your face and the odd grey hair.

Age will affect certain aspects of your life. It will have a bearing on your personal relationships; your role in the family will change; and so probably will your income. But there is no need to feel old in yourself. As soon as you begin to think in terms of 'three score years and ten', or, 'it's the wrong end of my life', it certainly is the wrong end. You have stopped living. Why assume that your best days are over? It is the future that counts and it could be long and exciting. I believe in looking forward. Think of all the wonderful things that are happening in modern medical science, and the fantastic recoveries people make which would have been unheard of not so many years ago. We are going to live longer if research goes on at the present pace. This is always provided, of course, that we keep ourselves as fit as we possibly can. Yet some people dwell on their little aches and pains and talk about them a bit too much!

Depression, grief, loneliness and emotional problems can make you weak, but you've got to bounce back or go under. The answer is not in the larder or the refrigerator. It is useless to pay nocturnal visits to the kitchen to help a hopeless love-affair. That will only make you more miserable and more concerned about your appearance, which is not the way to get a man or whatever your heart desires. You need confidence and fitness to do battle. If you are jealous, if some wretched rival is scratch, scratch, scratching at your happiness, you don't want to be fat and self-conscious.

Snap out of it

Well, what can one do to lift depression? There is only one answer, snap out of it. But how, you say, how? Well, even if the cause of the gloom is small, it is still the cause, so treat it first. If it's your hair, shampoo it or get it done. Having it cut is better still and can be a real gloom-lifter! If you cannot forget the longed-for telephone call, do the telephoning yourself.

Then do something different. Get rid of the rubbish (there is usually something you have always wanted to throw away) or clear the garden. Have a rest, feet higher than your head – it helps boredom and tiredness, I find. Breathe deeply to reduce tension or anxiety. Best of all, turn on the music and move. Exercise. It's astonishing how pepping up the circulation changes your mood. Tackle the gloom and let in some light. Build up your ego. You are a jolly nice person and completely original – there is no one just like you. Make a fuss of yourself if there isn't someone else around to do it for you!

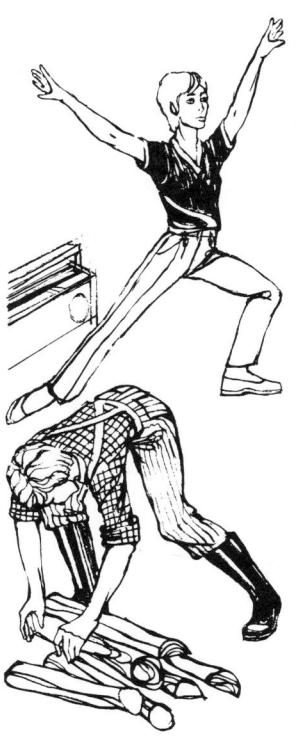

Work may not be the complete panacea for everyone, but it takes you a long way towards a satisfying life. Most work is creative; if you only paint the gate, you have created something which will give pleasure to others as well as yourself. Rusting iron is utterly depressing, but a new shiny black gate gives you a lift every time you see it. All right, it's work, and maybe a bit hard on the back or knees, but it makes you conscious of a few slack muscles you didn't know about!

Although I can never remember the Latin names of plants and marvel at those who do, I must say that I enjoy watching gardening programmes on television. I want to leap out of my chair and grab the nearest fork. Gardening is 'work' that is good for the figure and the mind. Naturally, all that bending, twisting

Kneeling
Sit back on heels to tighten thigh muscles.

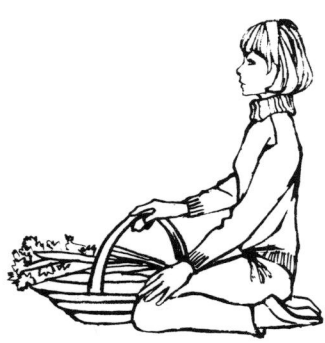

and stretching helps to firm your muscles, but it must be done the right way. If you go on weeding for too long when you are not used to it, an aching back defeats your enthusiasm and leaves you weary and worn. Working against time is another mistake. I find that the best way to benefit from gardening is to take time off and not worry about the clock.

Use gardening as a keep fit exercise. Never bend down with straight knees as the lower back suffers. Always bend the knees and kneel when weeding or planting. (A rubber mat is a good idea as it saves the knees and keeps them dry, and is obviously advisable if you have to twist.) During any rests, sit back on your heels. This is a wonderful exercise for the thighs as it tightens up the muscles. Sitting back may not come easily at first but it will with practice.

Reaching up to tie a creeper, or doing anything way above your head will be a good stretch for the waistline. Remember to bend your knees when picking up heavy seed boxes, flower pots, or a full watering can.

Breathe deeply while you are out in the fresh air – and you should soon feel that it's a great life.

Playing truant

Playing truant is another gloom-lifter. If you know perfectly well that you should tackle a particular job but the very thought of it makes you feel slightly sick, don't do it. It only makes things worse. The sickness is really fear. The best thing to do is to get out of the house. Go for a walk, tackle the garden, do anything that is active and in the fresh air. Do something that you like doing. Relax first – then tackle the job.

It is difficult for the dedicated and conscientious to relax in this way. I suppose our subconscious has a guilt complex and finds every reason why we should not do what we really want to do. It takes confidence to throw off the reins now and then, to down tools, slam the door behind you and rush outside. But you don't feel cheated – only glad you escaped.

Men seem to be better at playing truant than women. They are more objective and definite in their outlook. Sometimes what a woman may want sounds a little crazy (like walking in the rain just because the four walls have got her down). I say, put on your raincoat and put your best foot forward. It's our life; it's our cure for the doldrums. If we take care of ourselves we are better able to take care of others.

I am not suggesting that you follow a selfish existence – far from it. But I do believe that no one should be a slave to a guilt complex.

Thinking time

It has been my experience that a lot of people need to be left alone for a bit to give them thinking time. So often we feel too much and get emotional about situations which really require uninterrupted thought. 'Feel less and think more' is a great maxim and you don't have to sit and think. Sometimes an automatic movement of the hands helps – or something a little more active. Activities such as cutting the hedge, cleaning the car or ironing handkerchiefs release the mind to work out a problem more easily. Perhaps you will decide to sleep on it or perhaps you will do something about it now, even if it frightens you. I have known a telephone call made on the instant save a world of worry, and a letter written but not posted leave me thankful for days. Constructive thought and the time to analyse the pros and cons by yourself can unravel the tangles.

The importance of change

Everyone needs a change. Going on and on in the same old way can get very depressing and we don't always realise that we are bored with doing the same things at the same time every day, bored with living in the same surroundings, and bored with our appearance. Managing to change the scene when you feel like it is a real tonic; if you can't, try to change something else. There is nothing so ageing as being averse to change. If the change is wrong, well at least you tried it and confirmed that the old way suited you best. The main thing is to keep an open mind and to give a new idea a chance. It may make life look a little brighter. In many cases the best change of all is to lose weight, to make yourself fit and full of energy. The difference in the way you look and feel can change your whole outlook.

Overweight

A large percentage of the population of the Western world is overweight. Some people with many pounds to spare like the way they look, and because they are happy about their current shape accept some extra weight with grace and good humour. They are often delightful and lovable people. You have to accept yourself and love yourself if you want to accept and love others. Nevertheless, to be overweight is not healthy and can cause such illnesses as backache, varicose veins, arthritis, digestive and metabolic disorders, and can even lead to stroke, coronary and thrombosis.

The great majority of people, however, are frustrated by their inability to slim. They know that to carry so much weight around is potentially dangerous, and they realise that they are putting an unnecessary strain on the heart, and that problems of high blood pressure, arthritis and disease are more than a mere possibility. They tire more easily and are dissatisfied with their appearance. They will tell you that they really eat very little, so it cannot be food. Or they are downright honest and say that they cannot resist the dishes they love.

The problems of overweight are the same for men and women, so what are the reasons for compulsive eating? There are so many. It could be a habit from childhood (much overeating starts this way), it could be a form of escapism when things have gone wrong, comfort in emotional stress, or simply the result of being too good a cook. But whether the tendencies are inherited or acquired, indulging one's love of food can be extremely dangerous. It is so insidious. Unless there is a history of overweight or a medical cause, the first signs are a spreading waistline, wider hips and swelling thighs, the stomach protrudes and one is faced with the prospect of a double chin. How did it happen? Possibly because it was not noticed soon enough that the needle on the scales was going up steadily. Not everyone weighs himself regularly, and the extra two or three pounds mount up to stones over the years.

A definite danger period for putting on weight is later in life when we may harbour a conviction that the time for excitement, adventure and romance has gone, and we allow food to become a compensation. As people approach their forties and fifties they tend to take more interest in food and less in exercise. Take a look around you at your family and friends and you'll see what I mean. No longer the walk after the evening meal. There's something you want to see on television, and anyway there's a car outside if you must go out. Our friends – bless them – ask us to dinner remembering all our favourite dishes and little weaknesses. What can you say? Just smile and thank them – and slide a little further forward on the bathroom scales?

But bodies get even. They have their own ways of paying us back, making us know if we have offended. Indigestion, headaches, and a bloated feeling leave us in no doubt that discretion would have left us healthier and a little slimmer.

I think there are psychological dangers too in eating unwisely, particularly when rolls of fatty tissue attack and overtake an erstwhile lovely figure. It can be devastating and terribly depressing. Just one more reason why healthy slimming is a must. Do something about it now.

Taking action

What can we do about being overweight? For some, diet is the answer, making delectable dishes low in calories. Others cut out completely bread, potatoes and alcohol from their diet and lose pounds. Then there are the drastic dieters whom you meet one day in the street and don't recognise. Group therapy, weight lifting, health farms – there seems to be no end to the various ways to stay slim. The battle against the fat goes on, made worse by our friends on the sidelines laughing because their weight is constant and they can eat anything. Could it be that their metabolic rate is higher than ours and they are spared all the would-be bulges which cling to us? Until there is a real breakthrough in slimming research, we must press on ourselves, trying perhaps to find yet another way to win.

Take a good look at yourself in a long mirror, with nobody near enough to say, 'What are you worrying about? I like you that way – you are so cuddly!' But what matters is do *you* like yourself that way? Because in five years' time you won't be just cuddly, you'll be overweight. Figures don't stay the way you want them. In most cases, they tend to thicken and get set as the years go by, and only sensible eating and exercise can win the battle against time. But it's not easy to keep trim, especially for men. Giving up smoking, business worries, heavy lunches, or simply not enough time to keep fit makes it very difficult to keep the figure under control. It is just at this time in life when a young and slim appearance is such an advantage, too. No one can be forced into doing a bit of good for themselves, but you can persuade, drop hints, and quietly nudge your partner along the right road, and what better example to give than yourself?

I think the answer to overweight lies within ourselves. Do we want to keep reasonably slim, healthy and energetic, fit for what we have to do and want to do, or is the price too high to pay? It is as simple as that. I believe that we can achieve anything within reason if we make up our minds that it is all worthwhile. I wouldn't dare say that I have the right idea for every man, woman and child, but it works for me and my husband. I cherish my bathroom scale. I fuss it, and consult it twice a week. In this way I know to an ounce what is happening. If that needle rockets up even a pound, I'm on my guard, and I eat less until it comes down.

Keep fit food

Time and again I am asked if I diet. I don't. I find that what I term 'keep fit food' will keep me slim and fit at the same time.

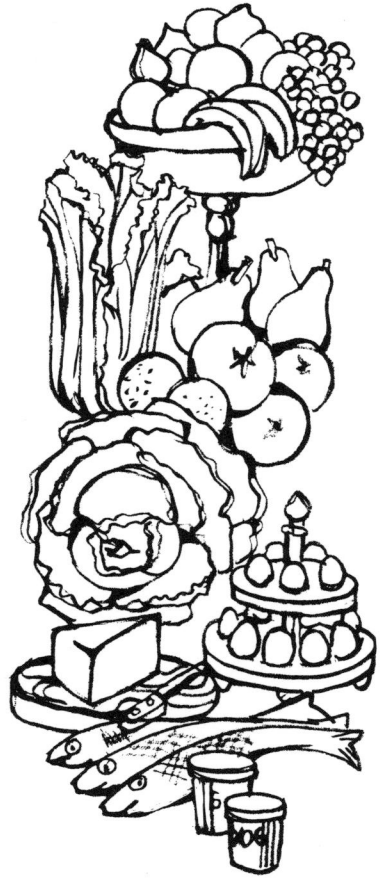

Junk, fatty and sugary foods quickly lose their appeal when replaced by meals from mainly natural sources. Natural foods and high fibre foods enable one to work hard with no fear of tiredness due to lack of proper nutrition, and they supply all the basic needs without putting on weight. The dishes are simple to make and require little cooking. It is a satisfying and enjoyable way of eating, and for the sake of both health and figure, well worth a try.

To my mind, it is far better to settle on a basic diet which you can follow as a way of life than to persist in eating all the wrong foods and then having to resort to crash diets. It is much safer and more becoming to lose pounds slowly and steadily than to lose weight suddenly. Most crash dieters swing between temptation and deprivation; they are always seeking a new way to slim, but seldom are they very happy about it.

If you need to lose several stones quickly for health reasons, then group therapy has a great deal to offer. At the weekly meetings, an expert lecturer will ensure that you don't choose the wrong diet. It may take longer to slim my way, but once you realise the value of the diet and accept it and enjoy it, it is there for the rest of your life.

High fibre diet

Scientists and researchers have discovered that in countries where there is a large intake of high fibre foods, few people experience the ills we suffer in the West. They have also noted that our soft and depleted diet can lead to cardiovascular problems, high blood pressure, abdominal troubles and cancer. There is already a big swing back to foods which have not been refined, or robbed of their original natural content.

The following suggestions for keep fit meals include dishes which contain a large amount of fibre.

Breakfast

1. Muesli or bran cereal or shredded wheat, with top of the milk, 1 teaspoon brown sugar.
2. 1 or 2 slices wholemeal toast, margarine. Boiled egg.
3. Grilled lean bacon rasher. Egg, scrambled or dry-fried.
4. Dried apricots, stewed.
Brown toast, margarine.
5. Fresh fruit – pear, apple or banana.
Brown toast, margarine.
6. Poached egg on toast.

46

Lunch
1. Welsh rarebit with grilled tomato.
   Black cherry or fruit yoghurt.
2. Brown bread and cheese with sticks of raw celery.
   Apple or banana.
3. Baked beans on brown toast.
   Stewed apple and honey.
4. Hard-boiled egg salad with lettuce, cucumber or
   mustard and cress and radishes.
   Fresh fruit.
6. Tomatoes on toast.
   Yoghurt.

Dinner
1. Chicken and green salad with home-made French
   dressing or lemon juice, or vegetables.
   Fresh fruit salad with honey.
2. Tongue with mixed salad or vegetables.
   Baked egg custard, with sultanas.
3. Liver and lean rasher of bacon, dry-fried or grilled,
   with tomato and peas.
   Fresh fruit salad.
4. Hard-boiled egg and cheese salad.
   Brown rice pudding.
5. Fresh cod or white fish, baked in a little milk with
   tomatoes, grated cheese and tomato sauce.
   Stewed apple.
6. Honey roast ham with mixed salad or vegetables.
   Yoghurt.
7. Cold lamb or beef with cauliflower topped with cheese
   and jacket potato.

Drinks
Weak coffee or tea.
Small quantities of sherry or wine.
Milk with cream crackers as a snack.

Important points
No deep-fried food.
No cakes or sweet biscuits.
No pastry or sweet puddings.
No sweets – occasional ice cream allowed.
No salt – except with egg or in cooking.

Always buy your salad ingredients, vegetables and fruit daily because the vitamin content is higher in fresh foods. If supplementary vitamins are required, it is sensible to take a multivitamin pill each day or pills containing Vitamins B and C.

Vitamin chart

Vitamin A
For growth, vision, maintenance of tissue, health of teeth, skin and digestive tracts. *Found in*: milk products, eggs, spinach, beans, carrots, lettuce.

Vitamin B complex
For maintenance of a healthy nervous system; essential for many bodily functions. *Found in*: milk, yeast, liver, kidneys, fish, eggs, vegetables, lean meat, fresh fruit.

Vitamin C
Defence against infection and stress; for blood building, healing of tissues, dispersal of fatty acids. *Found in*: citrus fruits, tomatoes and potatoes cooked in jackets.

Vitamin D
For bone development; important in growth and pregnancy; limited need by adults. *Found in*: sunlight, fish liver oils, fortified milk (i.e. milk with black treacle).

Exercise

Eating for health and a good figure is only half of the story. *Exercise* is the other half. It is the combination of the right food and enough exercise that will bring success to anyone who is prepared to follow the complete recipe. It is true that it takes a tremendous amount of exercise alone to slim you, but combine it with keep fit foods and you are away. You will find exercises and keep fit routines in the second half of this book, but don't forget that walking, cycling, swimming, jogging, cleaning the car, gardening and housework will also help to keep you slim.

Fortunately, energy usually returns with weight loss, and exercise is a must while the pounds are being shed. When you are fat, the stresses and strains are different and there are changes in posture due to the extra load. It is imperative to exercise regularly or the bad balance and posture which affects many overweight people will remain even when the weight has gone. Exercise will not only use up surplus fat and help the pounds to disappear, but if the muscles are toned up again as the body returns to normal, then the skin is less likely to sag. Sagging sometimes occurs when the skin has been stretched and muscles are slack.

There are occupational hazards, of course, for those who want to slim but whose jobs keep them chained to a chair or working long hours in a confined space or in a steamy kitchen (we cannot all choose our favourite work environment), but, generally speaking, if you follow my suggestions for healthy meals combined with plenty of regular exercise I am quite sure that you will beat any problem of overweight.

Slimming in the home

I won't pretend that I love housework but I do believe that it can be very good exercise. But is it enough to keep one supple and trim and to fine down the figure, or is that a fallacy? Of course, it all depends on how you go about it, whether you move well, and how much you do. It's like gardening. If you do too much at one time you'll end up exhausted. Plan it, and it can be very helpful. There are so many potential accident spots in the home that to tear round the house trying to do everything at once is very risky. If you really are terribly rushed, then the figure angle is unimportant, but if and when you have time to take things more easily you may find odd moments when you can do a few keep fit movements.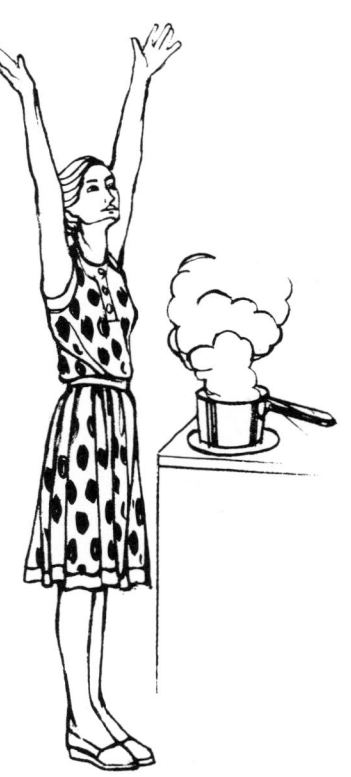

You can watch the milk, for instance, and stretch at the same time. Take both arms up sideways, and way above your head into a 'V'. Keep stretching and lifting the bust away from the hips. Rest, and stretch again. It's better than just standing there and slumping – or letting the milk boil over.

If you are using a vacuum cleaner, have your feet wide apart and follow it through as you sweep. This is quite a graceful movement. Switch it off and do one or two other exercises. Switch on the radio and find some music you can move to. This combination of housework and keep fit is a very good one.

Thousands of housebound keep fit enthusiasts have benefited by taking advantage of a little space and privacy. Even young children find exercising fun. But if, like one listener to one of my radio sessions, you decide to pick up something like a brush and swing it round in circles, please remember the lights. She hadn't got one left!

49

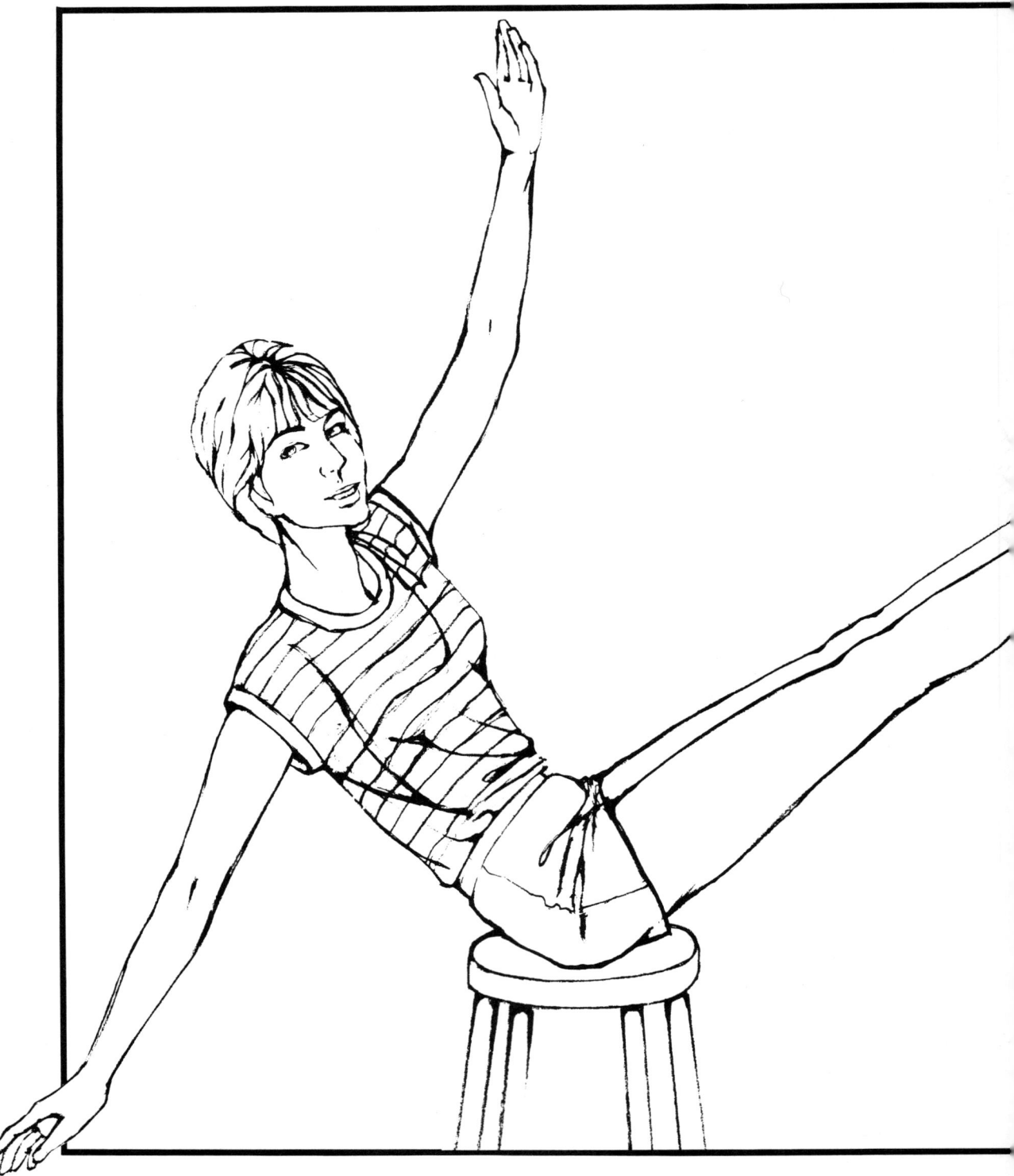

50

Chapter 5

Make yourself look attractive

**There is no real beauty where there is tension. Take care of the skin. The face has expression – a smile will lift lines in the face. Exercises for chin and neck. Keep shoulders and upper arms moving. Bustline basics. Arms, legs and thighs.
Don't take hands for granted. Foot and ankle problems can be avoided. Healthy eyes, teeth and hair.**

To a great extent, an attractive appearance depends on fitness. Everyone wants to look their best, and much of what I say in this chapter applies to both men and women. Basic requirements such as good posture and a good shape, vitality and a sense of well-being are catered for by following the six essentials described in Chapter 1. The finishing touches, however, come under the heading of good grooming, and it is this that can lift an average appearance into a class of its own. Good grooming can give a natural elegance which is not necessarily connected with the clothes we wear. It can give style and maybe a touch of glamour. It does not rely on expensive cosmetic preparations for its effect, but on time, thought and care.

Your face

Take your face, for instance. There is no real beauty where there is tension. Tension in the face is ageing but relaxation is youthful. It can smooth out lines in a face distorted by ugly tensions; it can change the whole appearance. Have you ever caught sight of yourself unexpectedly in a mirror when you were feeling bitter and angry? It was not your real face.

I think we have to be very conscious of what we are doing to ourselves and, however bad or tense we feel, we should try not to let it show too much. We must remember to relax our features or the lines we make will become permanent. The moment we let go and return to normal, the creases are ironed out and the face becomes harmonious and tranquil. I am not suggesting a poker face, far from it. A face full of expression is fascinating. Any lines we make should go up, not down. The laughter lines and any creases from smiling a lot simply do not matter, but the lines that habitually go downwards should be avoided. I am convinced that we line our faces ourselves. Concentration, worry and fear often take over when no one is looking, but just turn and smile at someone and the face softens. It is easy to talk, I know, and who cares about their face when really worried or scared. I am just saying that even when we are not miserable, we do not always bother to smile. So smile and say out loud 'I am beautiful – very beautiful,' and you will relax. Lines don't form overnight, and can be kept at bay for years if you relax your features.

Care of the skin
Be kind to your skin. Make sure that it doesn't get tired. Despite all the advice that goes with the millions of beauty preparations,

the experts still tell us that sleep is the best. What can you do with a tired skin day after day when it is deprived of enough rest? It becomes greyish in colour, sags and is ageing, and I know of nothing that really restores its freshness except sleep. Skin must be kept clinically clean. Nothing must clog the pores; a good herbal moisturiser helps, and make-up should be light.

Pollution is our enemy, particularly in towns and cities where particles of dust and dirt are everywhere. To counter the effects of pollution on the skin, it is important that as much leisure time as possible is spent in the fresh air in the right atmosphere so that the skin can breathe. Central heating can be another hazard. The heat builds up all day, and unless there is sufficient ventilation the skin suffers from dryness and dehydration. If you cannot turn down the heat, an open window is the only answer. Long hours of overheating, plus wintry winds, are very hard on the skin.

Lovely as it is, too much sunshine can also be harmful. Short sun-bathing sessions are fine – they make you look good and feel good – but to fry in the heat day after day dries up the complexion and encourages facial lines and wrinkles. I often wonder why sun-bathing is carried to such extremes. You have only to look at odd bits and pieces left on the beach and exposed to the sun, sea and wind to see what happens to them. Protection from these is very important for the eyes, hair and skin.

Excessive alcohol, strong coffee and smoking are other damaging factors, and if you value your skin they should be avoided.

If the skin tends to dry out then it needs help, and the solution can be very simple. I have never found anything better than a pad of cotton wool and a bottle of olive oil. This treatment removes make-up and keeps the skin soft; it doesn't feed, but it prevents excessive dryness which is the bane of many sensitive skins. It is slightly stickly, but a face flannel wrung out in warm water takes care of any surplus oil. Follow with plenty of moisturiser and, at night, a really good skin food.

Neckline and chin

So much for the face. The neck is even more important, and I must stress this. The face has expression – a smile will lift lines in the face – but not so the neck. It is an extremely youthful asset and should never be neglected.

The neck is not usually made up, so has no need of an oily cleanser, but a really good soap and loads of noisturiser and skin food works wonders. Massage well in, and up and over the jaw line, to help keep the contours tight and a double chin at bay.

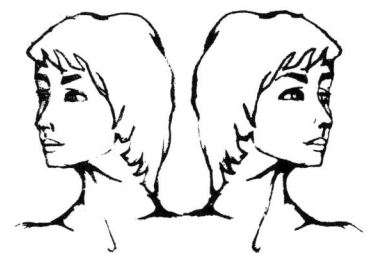

Head turning

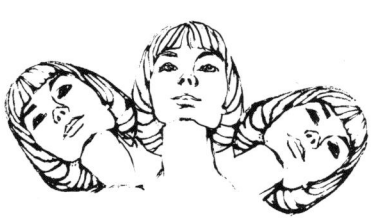

Head circling

It is essential to keep the head turning freely and to tone up the muscles of the throat. If the head is kept in one position for any length of time, the back of the neck at the top of the spine tends to become stiff and painful. If there is wear in the cervical vertebrae – and you can hear the slightest scrunchy noise when you turn your head from side to side – then I suggest that you do head turning exercises regularly and gently. It is imperative to loosen up the joints and keep them moving smoothly.

In addition to head turning, look up at the ceiling and high up round the room, then slowly circle the head in both directions. Apart from helping to keep a clean chin and jaw line, these slow movements have a relaxing effect. This effect can be heightened by gentle massage with the fingertips at the base of the skull. Massage where it hurts, and you will find that you will want to yawn and relax.

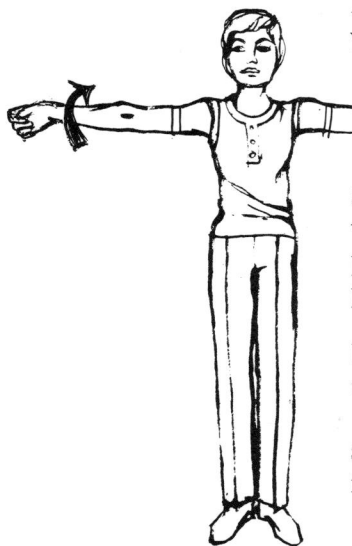

Skipping movement

Shoulders

Shapely shoulders and slim upper arms are a great asset and worth a little effort to maintain. They should be kept moving to prevent them getting set, thick or rounded. Shoulders are a focal point and need to be straight and supple.

Shrug the shoulders up and down and roll them round backwards in small circles. You will feel the top of the chest and upper back moving also.

For a stronger movement, with arms outstretched pretend to skip, circling the shoulders backwards to the count of eight. Circle for seven counts, then drop the arms and rest on eight.

Bustline

The bust is made up of glands and fatty tissue and it gets its support from the pectoral muscles in the chest, the firm skin, and, most important of all, good posture. Nothing is worse for a bustline than round shoulders. Shoulders and bust are inter-dependent, so while you are rolling your arms and shoulders backwards you are also lifting the bust.

If the bust is too large, then exercise can once again be combined with keep fit meals to help reduction. A lifted bustline is an integral part of a good figure, and you will find many movements in Chapters 9 to 18 which have a definite emphasis on the upper part of the body. It should also be remembered that a trimmer waistline will improve the bustline by contrast.

The three other basics I would advise for a good bustline are to wear a support bra properly fitted for added firmness, to splash the breasts with cool water at the end of a bath or shower to firm them, and to breathe more deeply.

Finally, I must repeat the advice of all medical experts, and this is to check the breasts regularly for a change of any sort. Look for trouble. Don't panic if you do find a lump. An early diagnosis will either put the mind at rest or be the quickest way to a complete cure.

Arms

While most men are quite happy with strong muscular arms, women demand a good deal of these useful appendages. Of course, they have to be strong for all the lifting and carrying women have to do, but, in addition, they need to be gently rounded, a nice colour – tanned or beautifully white – soft skinned and, above all, firm from shoulder to wrist.

A woman's pet aversion is a flabby upper arm with a handful of loose flesh hanging beneath, and if it happens to her own arms they are quickly covered up with long sleeves. The flabby upper arm problem usually arises when the person is overweight, or when weight reduction has been too fast due to crash dieting. Extensive slimming is less likely to cause the skin to remain stretched and loose in young people than it will in more mature women. Young skin usually tightens up again, particularly if the slimmer has exercised while losing weight. In middle age it is more difficult; the skin is not so resilient; it loses tone and, without its former padding, drops down. This is one of the many reasons why I believe in the benefits of slow slimming – unless fast weight-loss is imperative for health reasons.

Let us look again at the advantages of changing over to a keep fit way of life and see what the right food and exercise can do to improve the shape of the arms. I have to say that you should start to follow this regime as early as you can. Eat the right food and take exercise. Forget about any unsightly flab and use your arms. Bend them and stretch them and swing them. Play tennis, bowls, cricket, golf. Join in anything active, and never forget to twist your arms whenever you can.

A popular exercise for firming upper arms is called The Twist and it should be performed daily. Massage hand lotion into the skin to keep it soft and prevent a dry surface.

Stand with both arms outstretched at shoulder height, palms up. Twist arms and hands forward and round until the palm is

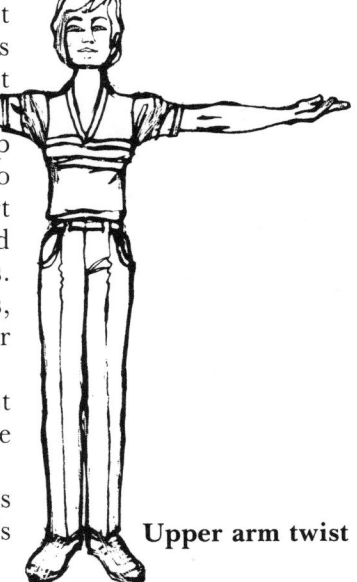

Upper arm twist

55

uppermost again, also the elbows. The shoulders will have followed the turn. Twist back to start and repeat seven times. Drop arms on the count of eight. Repeat, but do not overdo this exercise. Keep the movement firm but gentle.

If arms and elbows need a beauty treatment, then hand cream, a good loofah and half a lemon will keep them a good colour in winter. In summer, protect from the sun with a suntan lotion, and watch for burning. Flaking skin can be a problem and you should lubricate as much as possible if the skin is dry.

Legs and thighs

No one will deny that a good pair of legs is a great asset, and we can make them look longer and more attractive if we treat them well. Fortunately, good legs are by no means the prerogative of youth, and I have seen lovely legs on people well into their eighties. It is mainly a case of good bone formation, and if you have it, it can be made to last. If you do not have it, all the more reason to make the very best of what you do have.

Many women carry a great deal of their weight below the waistline, and there is often room for figure improvement in the area of the thighs. Heavy thighs can be caused by overweight or by heredity, and as many figures follow the family pattern, some so-called figure faults have to be accepted. However, I can only say that from my experience almost any figure improves with this slogan: 'Eat right, move more'. Get all the exercise you can – dance, cycle, run about, climb, play games – and use your legs.

The leg muscles will keep legs and thighs firm if they are made

Hip rotation
a Hold on firmly to back of chair. Lift outside leg, bringing toe across to touch floor in front.
b Keeping knee turned out and high, circle leg round towards back.
c Bring toe to floor, across and behind standing leg.

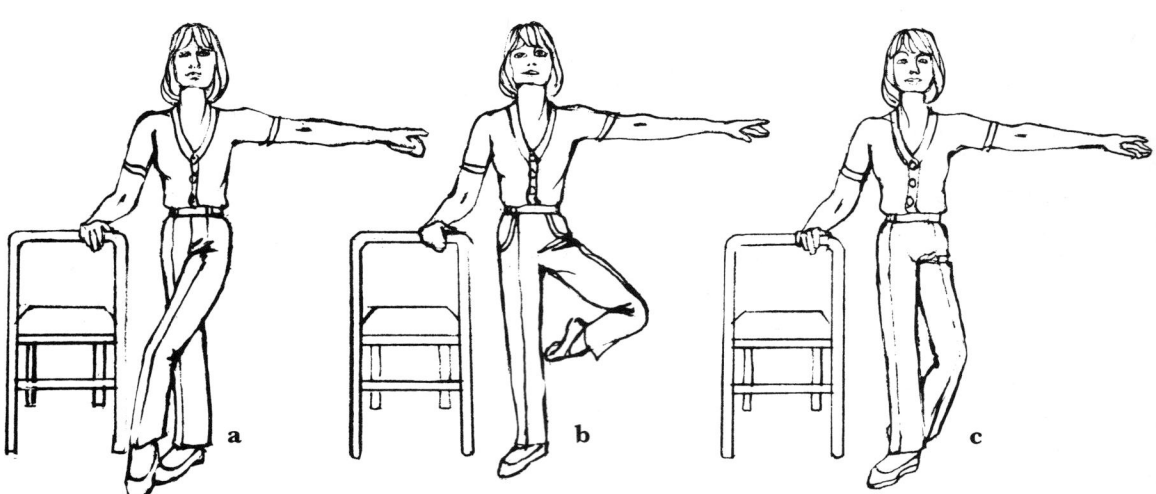

to work. They must be toned up, or they cannot give you the shape you want. Anywhere in the body, flabby muscles mean a flabby shape. At first, when you exercise there may be stiffness in knees and hips, but use the mechanics of walking to get supple again. Take big steps and feel the muscles making an effort. Always walk from the hips, never totter from the knees.

Pick out the leg movements from Chapters 9 to 18. Most of the movements are interrelated and your hips and seat will improve also. Put a hand on a worktop, table or sink and bend those knees; turn sideways and swing a leg to and fro. Do these exercises daily. Hand-cream your legs. Get them tanned naturally, if possible, or investigate a quicker way. Don't settle for a pair of white legs if any thread or varicose veins are present, but seek medical advice. Pull yourself up and away from your legs and don't let yourself settle down into your hips. Look for lunging exercises, as in fencing, and watch television sitting on your heels. All these are good thigh stretchers.

Remember that when legs are exercised vigorously there is a strong heart circulatory response, which makes leg exercises important for health.

Hands

Perhaps we take our hands too much for granted – I did, until the day I pulled the rockery to pieces. My hands were terribly painful as a result. It hurt to move even a finger, and it was agony to turn on a tap. Undue haste to finish an overdue gardening project led to strained muscles and ligaments – strain which could so easily have been avoided. My hands recovered quickly because I took my own medicine and gently exercised them every day in every spare moment. There is no doubt that exercise keeps the hands and fingers strong and supple and prevents the joints from stiffening. There are hand exercises in Chapter 7, and we often use these little movements in keep fit classes as a 'break' from the bigger ones.

Caring for your hands can be quite time-consuming, unless you have the type of skin which is impervious to dirt and hot water. A dry skin must be protected, so rubber gloves are a necessity for many household tasks. Hand cream should be kept close to the sink, and also half a lemon to remove any stain on the hands. If you have to search for gloves or cream, it is easy to forget to use them, but if they are within sight you should be able to keep your hands in good condition in spite of the chores.

If nails get rough and break easily, a hardening lotion applied to the tips does help, and the nails are better kept fairly short, using an emery board rather than a metal file. Standard methods of home manicure should do the rest, with perhaps professional attention every now and again.

Apart from regular care, it is equally important to relax the hands as tension frequently shows in them first. Fidgety and jarring little movements can be very irritating, and completely spoil the effect of good and careful grooming.

Feet and ankles

Many foot and ankle problems could be avoided if a few simple rules were applied to their care, and I think it helps to keep some of the possible hazards in mind. Many problems are caused by too tight or too short shoes, very high heels, narrow straps, and pointed toes. When the body weight is pushed forward on to the toes, they tend to curl under, or the subsequent pressure forces big toe joints out of line. Skin quickly hardens and leads to corns. In bad cases, ugly bunions form which cannot be removed without an operation. Ankles swell, and the resulting suffering shows in our faces. Other hazards include damp warm skin between the toes, which becomes itchy and infected, and ingrowing toenails, painful beyond words.

A well-fitting shoe is worth every penny; when fitting, allow room for heat and swelling, even if it means buying a slightly larger size. This applies to tights, stockings and socks as well. They should never restrict the foot. Whenever possible, walk barefooted to strengthen the muscles and ligaments in the feet and sit and exercise them as shown in Chapter 18. Efficient drying and powdering between the toes is essential, and so is cutting the nails straight across to avoid ingrowing. Remove dead hard skin with a special light foot file to help keep the feet comfortable. Soak feet and ankles in hot water and massage them gently with a simple hand lotion, and if your ankles swell, put your feet up. A light spirit or cologne will refresh them and if there is a problem, have a professional pedicure. Above all, don't wait until they hurt, take care of your feet now.

Feet and ankles
Sit on floor, hands at each side, feet together. Turn toes up as far as possible and then down to floor. Repeat gently several times.

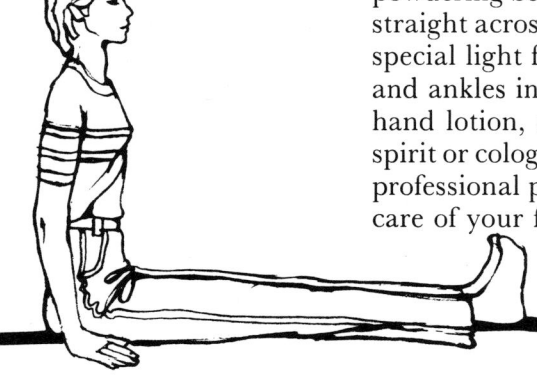

Eyes

Healthy eyes are a boon and a blessing and are sometimes taken for granted. It is often not until the telephone directory becomes slightly blurred that we begin to think seriously about their care. Eyes are subjected to a great deal of strain, but unless we are using them for close work day in and day out they will probably go along happily for years.

However, I still feel that a little extra care is well worthwhile, especially if your eyes get tired, irritate, dry out, water suddenly or hurt in a strong light. All of these things can happen even when the optician tells you that there is nothing fundamentally wrong and that the trouble is purely circumstantial or occupational. It is then up to you to sort out your own eye problems.

It pays to make sure that you work or read in really good light, coming preferably from over your shoulder. Regular eye checks are essential, as are really good glasses with attractive frames, or contact lenses, if you need them. Eyes need enough sleep to keep them from feeling and looking dull and tired. An eye bath used frequently will help them to sparkle. If dryness of the eyes is a problem, Vitamin A, found in fish oil capsules and green vegetables, will help the tear ducts to secrete their natural moisture. Parsley and spinach and vitamins B and C are thought to be good, too. Eating the right food solves so many of our fitness problems.

Never squint or strain in bright sunlight. Dark glasses, with a prescription built in for long or short sight, are far more comfortable and infinitely more becoming.

There are also eye exercises, which are excellent on waking. Try blinking, rolling the eyes round and round, looking to right and left, out to the distance and back to close up. You may remember being told to palm your eyes, cupping them in both hands, head down supported by elbows, until you can see only velvety black. This is very restful if they are feeling strained.

In times of real stress, there are excellent lotions, eye drops and a liquid type of cream which can get you out of trouble. Swimming in the sea is another aid. I'm sure the salt water helps my eyes.

Teeth

Most people show their teeth when they smile – and very attractive it is too when they are well kept and a good colour. I agree that they are often a lot of trouble coming and worse going but, real or false, they are too great an asset to neglect. Many teeth are lost early in life because the gums become diseased, and unless regular attention ensures that every particle of leftover food is removed there is a chance of the gums becoming soft and inflamed. Plaque builds up. Teeth are attacked by bacteria and eventually decay. They become loose and have to be taken out. To a great extent it is still our own dental care that decides the ultimate fate of our teeth.

These days we are encouraged to keep our own teeth for a lifetime, and we can if we look after them. Few people enjoy a dental session, but if they have been taken to the dentist often enough in childhood, they will usually continue to go regularly for check-ups. The trouble starts when there is no painful warning and the visit to a dentist is considered unnecessary. It may then be too late for even a multitude of stoppings. I knew of a case where a man developed what he thought was arthritis – he could hardly move a limb without pain. Subsequently, the real cause of the trouble was diagnosed and all his teeth were removed. He recovered almost immediately as the poison left his body.

Both for health and good looks, teeth are very, very important. They show. Tooth brushes should be renewed regularly and used up and down the gums and teeth rather than always across the teeth. Brushes need to be firm but not too hard. Dental floss is extremely useful for keeping the teeth free of decaying food pieces, and proper wooden tooth-picks are sometimes easier to use than floss for the back teeth. For an excellent mouth wash and colour lightener, use volume 10 or 20 peroxide, diluting one part peroxide to an equal part water.

If gums have become poisoned or inflamed, a hot salt water rinse will help in the short-term. Whatever the problem, cosmetic dentistry is now so advanced that when the time comes to replace your own teeth by capping or dentures, more often than not your looks are actually improved!

Hair

It is surprising that in these days of advanced techniques, many of us still find that looking after our own hair is a problem. Maybe it is because there are so many processes to choose from. Some can be very successful, but you do need a really good hairdresser, and in the end it all comes back to the condition of your hair.

The state of your health can affect the condition of your hair, and what you eat is more beneficial than anything put on the hair itself – only the roots are alive. If you are fit you have a better chance of having a lustrous head of hair than if you are overtired and tense. A nutritional diet consisting mainly of uncooked food, low in starch and fat, is said to be helpful in the maintenance of a good head of hair, causing less greyness and less fall out. Brewers' yeast contains the necessary vitamins, and sea foods are also specially recommended if you need supplementary help.

The editor of a famous national newspaper once told me that he owed his shining cap of fair hair to his mother's advice. 'Your job will make you tense,' she said, 'so every day massage your scalp from the ears upwards at the back of your head, then upwards from the front. Do not scratch your scalp but use your finger pads to move the skin until you feel it loosening up. It will stimulate the hair growth and help you to relax.'

I am convinced that this is excellent advice, particularly when the hair is dry. It distributes the natural oil from the roots to the ends, and certainly helps the hair to shine. A mild shampoo and conditioner also helps with shine, and a vinegar rinse can take care of hair which tends to tangle. Many people with dry hair like to use a shampoo made up of two egg yolks and a little shampoo to encourage lather.

Permanent hair colouring, bleaching and tight perming puts even a good head of hair at risk, as does blow-drying with too much heat or with the drier held too close to the head. Any hair which has been chemically treated needs care. Too much sunshine, chlorinated water or swimming in the sea without a cap can leave the hair very dry; it should always be protected to preserve its condition. If the hair is damaged it will dry out and will split. The only solution is to cut the hair frequently and allow the damage to grow out.

Condition is the word we should always bear in mind, and especially with day-to-day care. Hair brushes often feel sharp to the hand and can damage fine hair. The ends should be rounded, never spiked. Brushing regularly removes dust and stimulates the scalp, but it should not be carried on for too long unless the hair is very strong.

Central heating tends to dry the hair, as do strong winds and dust from the roads. If your hair is dry, this is where my old friend olive oil comes in. Before a shampoo, the hair should be parted all over the head and the oil rubbed into the scalp. Wring out a towel in very hot water and wrap it tightly round the head. After about ten minutes, when the warmth goes, shampoo thoroughly and rinse, finishing with a vinegar or lemon juice rinse.

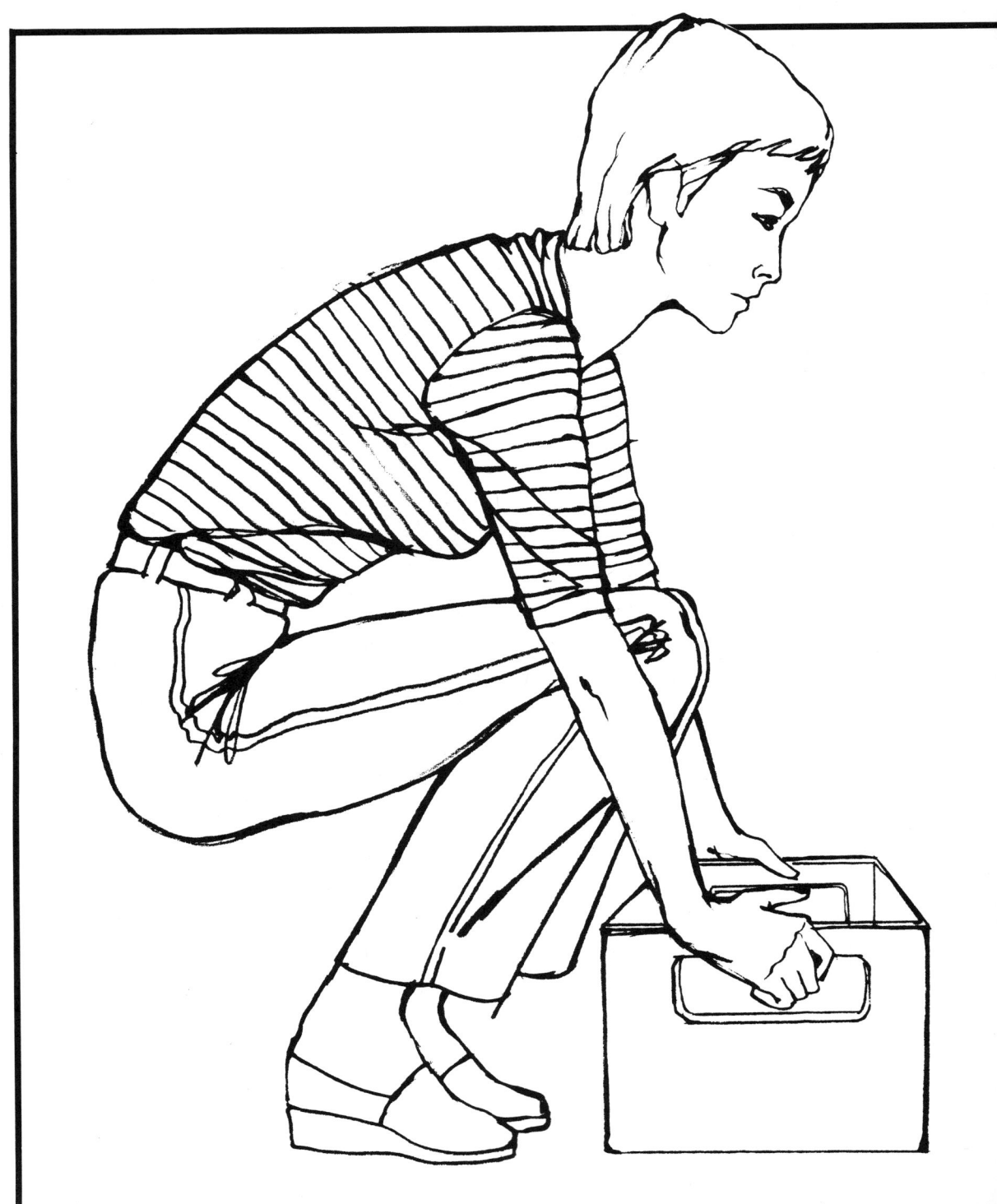

Chapter 6

Bad backs

My wish for a super spine. Intermittent and prolonged backache. Touching your toes and bending your knees. A firm bed. Accept that your back needs care. Stand tall and walk tall. Overweight people often have trouble with their backs. Housework and back strain. Backache in the menopause. Exercises to relieve the pain.

If I had three wishes, one of them would be for a super spine – a backbone so strong and flexible that in no circumstances would it ever ache! It is said that backache is so prevalent today that every year thousands of working hours are lost because of it. If this is true, why? Has backache always been a problem? I would think so. 'Mind your back' is a phrase which has its roots in truth. But do we mind our backs? The answer is no, not always.

Medical opinion supports the theory that much back trouble stems from postural faults, and that in many cases our way of life is responsible. We are told that some backache could be avoided if we were to hold ourselves correctly, if we were to stand tall instead of slumping, and sit with the base of our spine supported. We are told that we would suffer less if we were to strengthen our muscles with regular exercise and keep our joints free and mobile with more activity. We should also avoid long bouts of tension and improve our sleeping pattern. In short, we should consider our backs a great deal more than we do and treat them with care. This does not mean that our aching spines are unhealthy, but that we subject them to unnecessary strain.

In view of this advice, I think it is well worth while taking a look at backache and the daily hazards, seeing how we can avoid them, and, if they are occupational, see how they can be lessened.

Backache

A great deal of back pain is intermittent and due to any one of many causes. If backs are treated with care, the vast majority of them should be able to support our various movements without any problem. Backs like to be used in a free and relaxed manner and their enemy is sustained tension. The spine needs to be flexible and mobile, and the supporting muscles strong and able to stretch and relax as required.

Overcoming intermittent backache is a question of maintaining the muscles and ligaments of the back in good order, with exercise, so that they can recover naturally. A handful of good movements properly learnt and carried out each day can keep backache at bay. However, if backache is prolonged it should be investigated and diagnosed as soon as possible. Investigation is imperative as the pain might be secondary to another complaint.

If the pain is due to injury or is becoming chronic, seek the advice and treatment of an osteopath. His specialised knowledge and experience, coupled with years of training, is invaluable and sometimes he can get you out of pain immediately. I have seen manipulation that looks like a miracle. Alternative medicine, like orthodox medicine, does have a place. Some people find acupuncture helpful too.

Severe cases of spinal injury are usually placed in the hands of orthopaedic surgeons and doctors, probably necessitating weeks of hospital treatment, bed rest and access to X-ray equipment.

Daily hazards

Bending the knees

Picking things up incorrectly is a common cause of backache. When we bend forward and go down with straight knees to touch our toes as many people still do, we put a great strain on the lower back. We must *bend* our knees, and let the legs take the strain.

I have always thought that there should be posters on every hoarding saying, 'Let your legs save your back.' This may sound a little odd but, believe me, it is basic common sense. You would be surprised at the number of men and women who say to me, 'I'm all right, I can touch my toes.' And down they go, there and then, with straight knees and often put both hands flat on the floor in front of them. The loose-backed ones – the double jointed, the acrobatic – don't seem to suffer, but most people do.

Bending with straight legs puts a great strain on the back. An orthopaedic consultant once said to me, 'Bad backs are all your fault.' 'My fault?' I said indignantly. 'Whatever do you mean?' He said, 'I'm very tall, as you can see, and at school I was forced to try to touch my toes and I was actually banged on the back by the teacher. I have never recovered.' It took me some time to explain to the consultant and several amused nurses that all this 'touch toes' business went out with the Flood. For twenty years or more

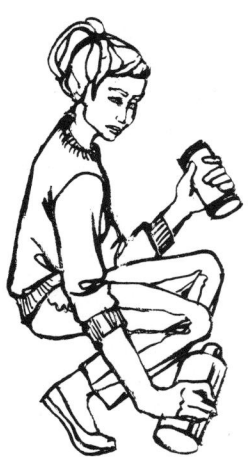

Lifting
If working or lifting at low levels, squatting and bending your knees will save your back.

To ease the back
Relax towards your toes, bending your knees. Uncurl and stand tall, leaving head until last.

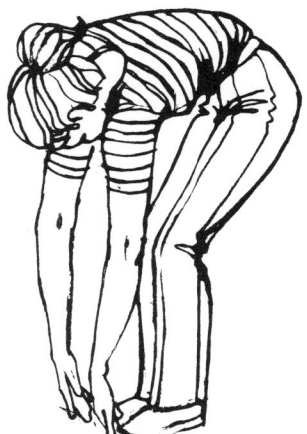

we have known that we had to teach people to bend their knees. Always bend the knees – don't just dive to the floor.

It is a mistake to make the back do all the work when the legs can help to take the strain. If you are lifting a heavy weight, go down with the back as straight as possible, feet slightly apart and close to it. Pick up the object, and push up with your leg muscles and the top of your head. Great care should be taken to think first and lift deliberately when lifting heavy weights from the floor. Hug the object; never lift anything heavy at arm's length.

As an exercise, the relaxed drop down of Rolling Pin Roll (Chapter 10) and the slow uncurling of the spine is a good movement to make the back more supple and to strengthen it. This is, of course, the modern way to touch the toes.

Sitting

This particular hazard is insidious. Most people have their favourite armchair and it is very pleasant to sink into its depths in order to relax after a long and tiring day. If your back is aching, *don't*. The armchair will only make it worse. And it is especially bad if you sit with your lower back inches away from the back of the chair and your legs stretched out on the floor in front of you.

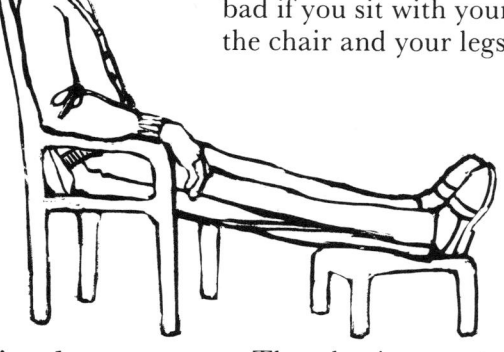

Armchair ache
Never sprawl or slump when sitting. Always sit firmly supported.

The classic way to sit is to forget about sinking into soft upholstery and to choose a firm chair that fits you. You will then be unable to slide forward. Slip a small hard cushion in the hollow of your back, or wherever you need support. Ideally your knees should be a little higher than your hips. If you can beg, borrow or steal the kind of footstool used by your grandmother, put your feet up on that. If you can get hold of a rocking chair, this is wonderfully soothing to the nerves.

If your back is really troublesome, lie on it – flat out on the floor. (I know someone who, since an accident, invariably watches television this way.) Sitting on the heels helps, and so does squatting, kneeling and any change of position. The objective is to prevent a build up of tension and to avoid the muscles going into spasm, because then the back will really hurt. Don't sit all evening. Get out of your chair to change the television programme. Ignore the remote control – get up and press the knob! To relieve a clamped-down feeling, stand up and stretch. My favourite stretching exercise is The Ladder (see Chapter 10).

Take the arms up sideways and climb an imaginary ladder – hand over hand, rung after rung. Do this several times with a short rest in between. The upward stretching helps to open up the vertebrae and prevents you from sinking down into your hips. Lolling in a chair encourages this sinking so the more you stretch the better. Never, never jerk while doing The Ladder, but make it a fluid upwards movement.

Driving a car for long hours without a break is hopeless if you have a bad back. Here again, the sitting position is very important. Some drivers lie almost flat out at the steering wheel, with one leg permanently stretched with the foot on the accelerator pedal. Far better for your back to pull the seat closer to the steering wheel so that the knees are higher than the hips. You may not agree with this at first, but try it. In traffic jams and while waiting for the lights to change, turn your head from side to side, shrug your shoulders and roll them backwards in small circles. These small exercises may amuse (or even frighten!) the driver behind you, but it will relieve any tension in the muscles. Stop at a lay-by on long journeys and stretch your legs. It may be a bore but these little breaks are kind to the body and leave you more refreshed on arrival.

A firm bed

An uncomfortable bed can cause back problems. The firmer the bed the better, provided it does not make all your bones ache. Both bed and mattress need to be in good condition for maximum support, and, if necessary, a board beneath the mattress will prevent any give.

Bedclothes, preferably a duvet, must be warm and light. Turning in bed under heavy tucked-in sheets and blankets which do not move with you can cause serious back trouble. Sleeping on either side is normally better than on your stomach or back, but if in pain ringing the changes does not always help.

If the pain is really bad while you are in bed, here is the advice given to me by an osteopath many years ago. Turn down the bedding, leaving a free space. Face your pillows (you will need

The seal
Lie like a seal on top of two pillows, for temporary relief from pain.

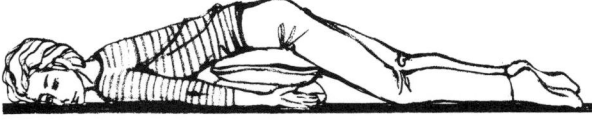

two) but be careful how you turn – don't twist. Kneel and slip both pillows under you where you feel the pain, then lie on top of them, face downwards like a seal, with your back higher than your head. It is not a comfortable position if held for very long, but it will stop the pain temporarily and give you a breather. Care must be taken when you handle the deadweight of the pillows.

Knowing your back

Accept that, however young and fit you are, your back needs care. A bad back can happen to you, and for the back that has worked hard all its life there is the problem of wear and tear. It is essential to avoid going on for too long at any one thing. As soon as the back becomes tired and begins to ache – *STOP*! If it is possible, lie down flat, preferably on a hard floor, and try to relax completely. Relaxation comes with practice (see Relaxation, Chapter 1).

Floor rest
Not an ideal sleeping position, but excellent floor rest for an aching back.

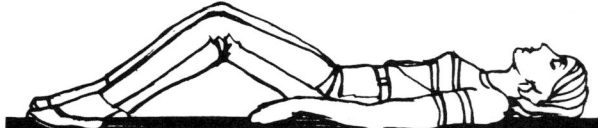

One of the most difficult problems for any of us to solve is how to separate our working programme from our leisure activities. Some of us have an inborn guilt complex – the inner voice which says, 'But you can't stop now,' and on we go until we are utterly exhausted. We have no enthusiasm left for that activity or rest we promised ourselves when the jobs were over. This is not what nature intended – and we are losing efficiency in the process.

I have the greatest admiration for the dentist who knows that most of his working life will be spent in an impossible standing position endeavouring to see further into his patients' mouths. The stresses and strains of his way of life must be enormous. An electrician I spoke to after he had worked for some hours in a cupboard half his height said that his backache was simply appalling. There are many such examples of occupational backache, and each is an open and shut case for exercise and rest, which is what our muscles need.

Hold your arm out with no support and see how long you can keep it there. Tension builds and you have to drop the arm and let it relax. This is what we have to do with ourselves. I believe that except in real emergencies we should not listen to our guilt complexes and as soon as we begin to feel tension mounting we should stop! Before we really begin to hurt. The tension will not get better until you take a rest. Frequent stops will prevent the utter exhaustion which eventually becomes an ache.

Before resuming a cramped position or a tiring job, give your muscles a change. Do a few mobilising movements – stretch, bend, circle, swing, kick and relax. Move more.

Weight

It is important to keep your weight at a reasonable level as many overweight people have trouble with their backs. Where there is excess weight it is usually carried around the stomach area and there is sometimes a tendency to arch the back to compensate. The body is pulled out of perfect alignment and is much more likely to become strained in the lumbar region. Then, if through lack of exercise the back is out of condition, lumbago becomes a possible hazard. Lumbago can also occur during pregnancy as the weight increases, but this is a medical problem and a doctor should be consulted. Nutrition comes into the picture too, because crash dieting can lead to a weak back – so eat the keep fit way.

When they are working, muscles need a much greater supply of blood and they need to relax in order to have this supply replenished. Life must be a mixture of work and rest, never working in sustained tension. If you are walking, running, swimming or dancing, these activities are energetic and without rest periods they do no good. Bending over a typewriter, carrying heavy bags, driving or lolling in a chair, anything fixed, has the opposite effect: keeping the neck, shoulders and back still for long periods subjects them to strain and they tire very easily, and to counteract sustained tension they must move.

We have been shown on television the wisdom of regular exercise routines which break up muscle tension, a system followed by factory workers in countries like Japan and China. A huge output is demanded in these factories where the workers have the most intricate jobs to do. Their output is doubled and trebled because they are instructed to move to music several times during the day, standing by their own particular work place. I have taught many factory workers in this country in their spare time, and have always hoped to see a similar plan of 'active rest' organised. It has, I believe, been done in some smaller British and Japanese-owned factories, but it would be a great step forward if exercises could be introduced generally. Postural strain and muscle fatigue can be avoided if routine is broken up by even small movements.

Exercise and deep massage help where there is fibrositis, for instance. It is useless to keep the area still, and rigidity must be avoided.

In the house

Many women complain, with good reason, about housework and the effect that some chores have on their backs. Using a heavy sweeper or very thick mop puts a jarring strain on the lower back. This strain will not be felt if you move around the room freely, always having one foot ahead of the other so that the whole body is on the move. The trouble comes if you stand with both feet together and just push back and forth with arms and back.

Ironing can be very wearing on the neck and shoulders unless you stand with your feet a little apart and let your weight shift from one foot to the other as you iron. See that the ironing board is at the right height so that you can work with a reasonably straight back and relaxed shoulders. Wear comfortable shoes with low heels, and trousers or a fairly full skirt if you have much to do; high heels push the weight over on to your toes, and a narrow skirt restricts the movement of hips and knees. Ironing is so tiring and restricting anyway that you need to be and to feel as free as possible as back fatigue and cramped shoulders reduce efficiency. Fortunately, these days fewer materials actually need to be ironed.

A long job at the sink or worktop can tire your back unless you stand with feet apart and change your weight, as with ironing. Standing at attention with feet close together is not advisable. The tension builds, just as it does with a soldier on sentry duty, and a tense spine will eventually ache.

I have noticed in my own case that unless I am in working clothes, I tend to lean away from the sink to protect the front of my dress, but at the same time my shoulders or arms go forward towards it. This is very bad for the back, and if you tend to do the same then keep an apron handy to tie on quickly so that you can stand straight all the time.

The menopause

One of the symptoms of the menopause, as with pre-menstrual problems, is an aching back. This is why I say to women, with my hand on my heart, follow the keep fit way of life. If the middle years find you fidgety, nervous, short tempered, tired, and with an aching back, then the fitter you are the better.

Being fit will mean that you will have a stronger back and your whole outlook will be one of confidence. You will be active and concerned with your daily exercise programme at home, or your regular weekly keep fit class. You will know how to relax so that you are not overtired; you will know how to allow time for sufficient sleep, and instead of possibly eating for compensation you will have adopted a sensible eating plan and therefore will have kept your figure and your looks.

It is not always the distress of the symptoms that upsets women if they suffer at this time, it is the way they allow themselves to look. Appearance is something that you can do something about. I mean this very seriously: start keeping fit now and you won't regret it. I promise you.

Posture

Whether your purpose is to help a bad back or to prevent one, the golden rule is to stand tall and straight. Measure up to a flat wall, as in Posture, Chapter 1. I say this because if you have had back pain it is possible that you are instinctively trying to get away from it and putting the weight in the wrong places. Maybe you have developed a habit of standing on one leg with the hip jutting out, or of slumping a bit in the middle, or perhaps the stresses and strains which have caused your backache have affected your stance in some other way. In each case, correction is vital. Do the posture correction exercise and, having stretched yourself into line, make a point of standing that way.

Always sit up straight in a chair, with the base of the spine supported by the back of the chair in the correct manner.

Walking tall is very important for bad backs – and for good ones too, for that matter. Low heels and empty arms are essential. Walk for pleasure whenever you can because once you start carrying heavy loads or wearing shoulder bags for any length of time, back will come the stresses and the strains. Walk for pleasure in your spare time, swinging along feeling weightless and free. Move smoothly from the hips. Be relaxed, because if you try too hard the tension will give you a stiff kind of gait. Let yourself come up to your full height as you go along, head held high.

An arched, or sway, back can be caused by wearing very high heels day after day. The wearer may be slim but the weight is thrown on to the toes, and straightening up the head and shoulders will produce a hollow in the back. You see this sometimes in a lesser ballet dancer, and in this case the seat usually protrudes as well. Apart from an ugly line, the risk of backache is great and if backache is already present then bad posture makes it very much worse. Wearing shoes with heels of varying heights – from flat up to two inches – is the safest way to guard against an aching back.

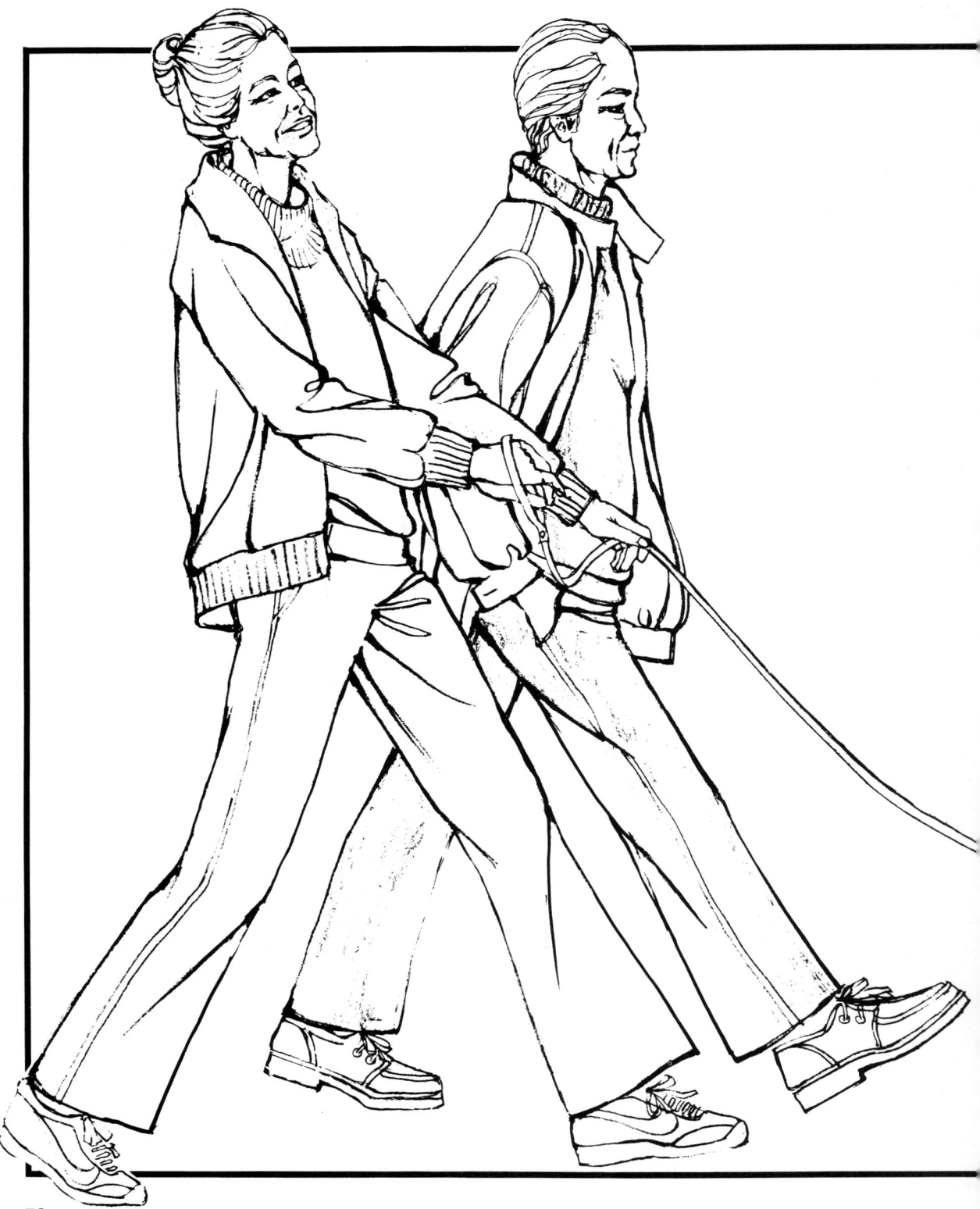

Chapter 7

Fit to retire

Fitness can be your fortune when it comes to
retirement. Welcome the extra hours of
active leisure. Plan and prepare. Don't let
retirement just happen to you. A shake-up is
stimulating. Enjoy yourself. Good circulation
has a great deal to do with longevity. Keep fit
so that age will have no meaning.
Selected exercises and mini movements.
Water therapy. Nutritional requirements.
Retirement reminders.

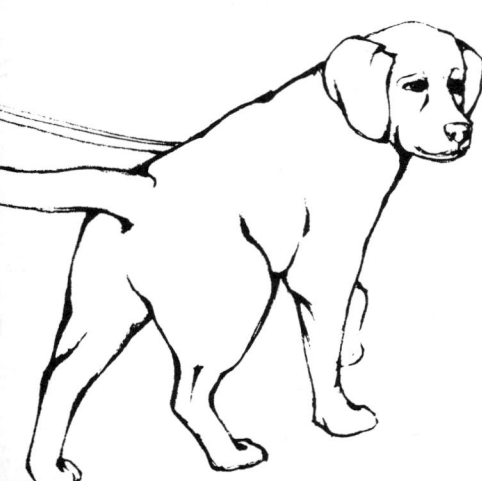

Fitness can be your fortune when it comes to retirement. It can smooth the way and make retirement a goal, instead of the finality that many people dread. If you already appreciate the enormous value of good health and are fit yourself, then you are off to a good start. You will continue to maintain that feeling of well-being throughout the coming year. You will not be worrying about how you will fill the extra time on your hands; you will know where you are going and welcome the extra hours of active leisure. If you wish, you will have the energy to work at something else or to use the skills you already have. If you are not as fit as you would like to be, here is the opportunity to build up your health.

I see retirement as a change for the better. Not since we were growing up have we had so much time to be out in the fresh air, free to walk when and where we will, free to cycle, to swim, to test our model trains, or to visit long-distance friends. A whole new world is opening up before us. Expensive? Not really. There are dozens of ways to get out and away at a reasonable cost. Usually someone we know has a car and the high cost of petrol can be shared between friends. You can travel by train for half the normal fare and local transport is either free or subsidised. Pride should not prevent anyone from using these facilities – or from claiming other benefits – after all, they have been earned.

Plan and prepare

Retirement may be years ahead for you and your family, but it is possible that in the future the specified age may be lower than it is today. Add to this the longer life expectancy and you have a situation where it might be wise to prepare for retirement now. As a well-known doctor remarked recently, 'Don't let retirement just happen to you. Think about it, look forward to it and plan.' He referred to our basic needs: somewhere to live, insurance policies to mature at between sixty and sixty-five, a medical nest egg, deciding what you can do and what you want to do, your health, and your attitude to the entire undertaking. If your attitude is to be one of disappointment, regretting the loss of status, identity, income and friends, then lack of preparation can make things worse. If the shock of retirement is suddenly thrust upon you, leaving a feeling of deep resentment, then life can seem empty and purposeless. Fortunately, for many people it is a longed-for change and their positive outlook accepts the challenge. If you have faced up to retirement and prepared for it to some degree, it is rather like making a will – make it and forget it. That is something else out of the way. Now we can get on with our lives.

A man I met recently told me that for years he had worked for an authority, and when one Wednesday he became sixty-five years of age he was not allowed to finish out the week. His colleagues bewailed his imminent departure. 'What shall we do without you?' they said. When he dropped in to thank them for their presents, they were completely disinterested. Shocked and bewildered he continued to rise early and was helpful about the house. Having always enjoyed growing roses, he moved to a village where he had a garden and there were many young people. He painted the village hall and became an 'Uncle' to all the children around.

So much for the man – fit as a fiddle, he was able to cope. His wife was less fortunate. Accustomed to less housework and more outings, she developed painful feet and knees and prepared herself mentally for a life with arthritis. Finally they settled for doing their own thing – to live as two good friends, to have individual interests. If one did not want to go out, the other did not feel obliged to stay in. The arrangement worked. When two people, used to normal daily separation suddenly have to spend every hour together, they may find out that they have no common interests.

Another fact of retirement was revealed to me when I questioned a lady I know quite well. I asked her how she had dealt with the problems. 'Problems, what problems?' she said. Feeling somewhat uncomfortable I explained that I knew of one difficult situation at least. Having arrived home for good, the husband became frustrated at having nothing to do and he missed his friends and responsibilities. He had been used to a life in management and he more or less took over the running of the house: he spent a good deal of time in the kitchen, did the shopping and expected his wife to watch television during the afternoon. 'What rubbish,' my friend said. 'People don't change. Retirement is merely an extension of their way of life. If they founder on the rock of retirement, they were never good sailors – the new adjustments simply found out the cracks. The wife should have known what to expect and should have been prepared for it.' And away she went.

Of course there will be problems. Not least the drop in income. Because so many people cannot envisage a standard of living other than the one to which they have become accustomed, they cling to their family houses and gardens, trying to deal with the rising costs of maintenance, forgetting that the do-it-yourself jobs become harder as the years go by. Far better, I think, to sell, buy something smaller and invest the rest of the money sensibly to augment the pension.

I believe in change. A shake-up is stimulating and makes you feel more vital and energetic. It provides other interests and you are less likely to grow old before your time! To bring real joy to your 'new life' you need to be as fit as you possibly can. Given reasonable health, this can be built up to a vitality and energy level that is normally associated with youth. Fitness at any age is largely a matter of common sense and looking after yourself.

If you don't take enough exercise, eat too much or too little, go short of sleep and fail to relax, then of course you will age and you will need that pension. But if you are determined to stay young, you will probably be able to add to it.

Enjoy yourself

I would like to see more attention paid to the enjoyment of retirement. If you begin to slow down in middle years this is no reason to assume that by the time you retire you will have to stop altogether. On the contrary, provided you realise that you are not quite as energetic as you were, retirement is just the chance you need to get going again. If you are really tired, then take things easily for a while and assess the situation. Maybe a holiday will renew your enthusiasm. When work has been your whole life, you don't always leave it without some regret. Give yourself a chance to look round and decide what is best for you now. Decide, whatever else you do, to enjoy yourself. This goes for everyone – married or single.

It is such a terrible mistake to take your pleasures sadly. I see so many people well supplied with all they need, but they are not happy. Surely, this is the moment to spread a little happiness and enjoy yourself at the same time. This truth was brought home to me in a recent telephone conversation I had with the chairman of a national organisation. A retired headmistress, she had turned her talents towards organising, advising and supporting a hundred good causes. She spreads her unlimited energy all around, and is happy and contented. There are many others like her. Get fit, stay fit and enjoy yourself.

So let us channel all the energy we can muster into being active for the rest of our lives. Of course, there are many people whose nervous energy will keep them going and they will never 'retire' in the usual sense of the word.

A sense of humour

A sense of humour is a great blessing at any age. I'm sure you've met the fantastic person who, crippled with arthritis, sits in his or her wheel-chair and keeps everyone in sight amused – and full of admiration. If I feel tired or my finger aches I am not amused. Oh, what a blessing is health – positive health that lets you jump out of bed and survey a new cold wet day as if it is filled with sunshine. That is something that needs a sense of humour to start with!

But there are people who can do this. I have met them in all walks of life and it really shakes me. It intrigues me. I want to know why. Here are people in their seventies, eighties and even nineties, who are active, smiling and filling every hour of the day doing something for somebody. Perhaps that is the answer, but they must be able to do it. Their minds and bodies must let them or they would be sitting quietly or have taken to their beds instead of keeping going. I am sure that the less you do, the less you want to do – and the more you do, the more you can do.

I cannot believe that, just because we are brainwashed at a certain age to think that our working life is over, we should take on the mantle of the old and sit back and watch the world go by. *Get out of that chair!* Anyone can sit down and say, 'Well, what can I do about it?' But apathy is insidious and can eventually pervade your whole life. Surely, retired people have something to offer those who have not yet lived long enough to know most of the answers? We have seen a lot of it happen before anyway, and experience can be very useful.

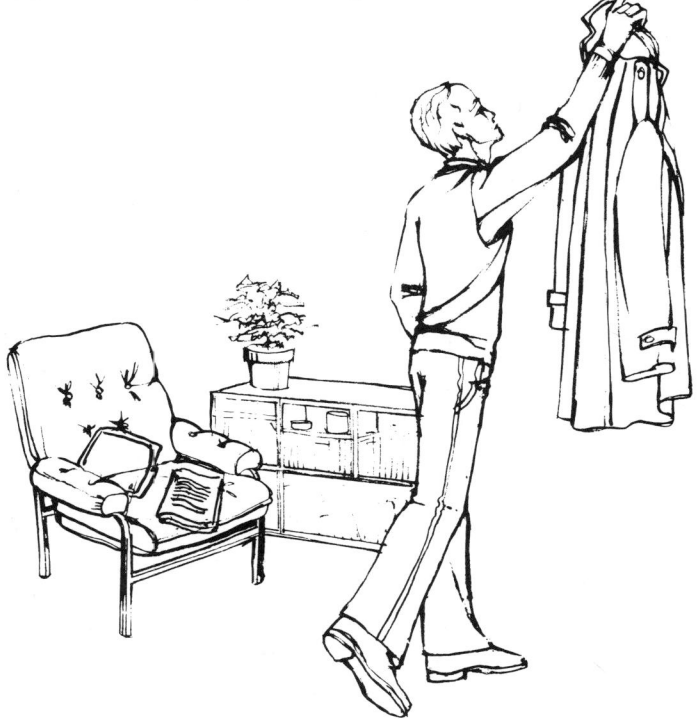

Exercises

Health is happiness

There is such a diversity of opinion where health and happiness are concerned that it is not easy to suggest the same fitness programme for everyone. However, if you agree with me that in most cases health is happiness, then we can start from there.

It is interesting to see how ideas differ on the subject of fresh air. At any age, some people will make for the nearest beach when on holiday; others will stop their car by the sea and wind down the windows. Some people will take a bus or a train and walk for miles; others will spend most of the day travelling by coach. The important point is that they are all getting out, changing the scene and putting variety into their lives, and variety is essential in retirement. To be bored is to be unhappy and leads to frustration and tension, so out we must go. If I have convinced you that it is fun to be fit, I would like to repeat that the six essentials I have written about in Chapter 1 are for everyone. They apply at every age and at every stage in our lives.

Retirement is the time to strengthen your muscles, to keep mobile, and to pep up your energy and circulation. Good circulation has a great deal to do with longevity and is essential for the health of mind and body. A few simple movements practised each day will help. They will also keep the skin looking younger, firmer and a better colour. Make a place in your daily life for these movements. If you have never before moved in this way, start now. We may retire from our main occupation, but we do not retire from life. If we keep ourselves fit, then age will have no meaning.

Check with the doctor

Men and women of retirement age who want to do my exercises but have a health problem of some kind should check with their doctor first to make sure that they are fit enough to do them.

If this type of exercise is completely new to you, start with the simple movements and leave the faster and more advanced routines until you are ready for them. As I shall not be teaching you personally, I have put together six exercises from different chapters which will gradually lead you into the more general routines. There is no merit to be gained from overdoing movements when you begin – you might feel stiff and be put off exercise for good. If you are of retirement age, these are your exercises. Please start gently.

Selected exercises

Chapter 10, exercise 1
The Ladder: For good posture and waistline

Stand tall, feet very slightly apart. Raise one arm up sideways close to head, then the other. In this position, stretch upwards towards the ceiling with alternate arms, as if climbing a ladder. Feel the stretch right through the body. Drop arms and relax.

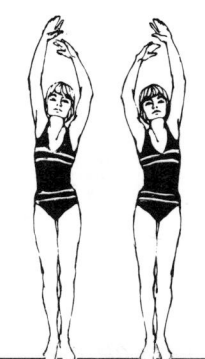

Chapter 16, exercise 4
Backstroke: For chest muscles, shoulders and upper back

Stand tall. Stretch one arm forward, upwards, round and down, making a complete circle. Do this slowly and strongly, as in the backstroke, keeping the arm close to the head on the upward stretch. Repeat with the other arm.

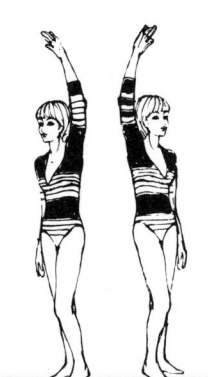

Chapter 14, exercise 6
Punch: For mobility and waistline

Feet well apart, knees relaxed and weight on right foot. Make a fist with right hand and, bending the elbow, twist to the left and punch. Repeat with the left arm, punch to the right.

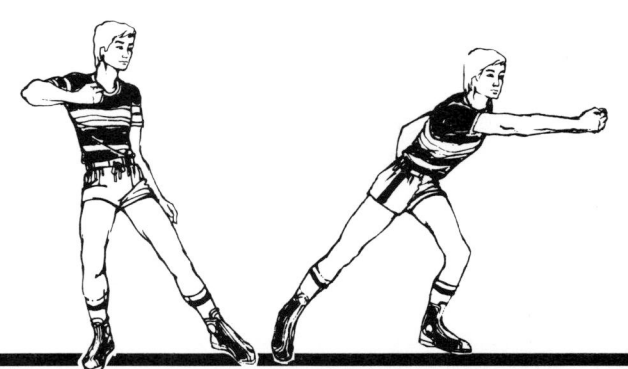

Chapter 11, exercises 4 and 3
Swingtime: For mobility and general toning

Feet well apart, knees relaxed. Let both arms swing across the body from side to side like a pendulum. Keep swinging, changing weight from foot to foot. Then swing high, looking up at arms and swing low towards feet, looking down and bending knees.

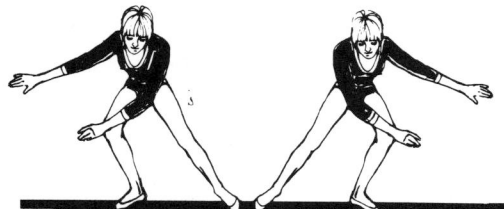

Chapter 10, exercise 2
Knee Clasp: To strengthen stomach muscles

Lie flat on floor with feet up on seat of a chair or low stool. Lift left leg, bend and clasp with both hands. Pull gently towards chest. Stretch and put down. Repeat with right leg. After practice try with both knees together. A cycling movement can be added.

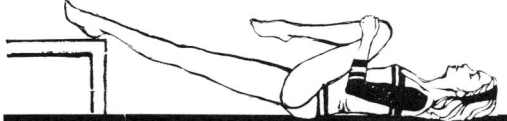

Relax and Stretch: For mobility and good posture

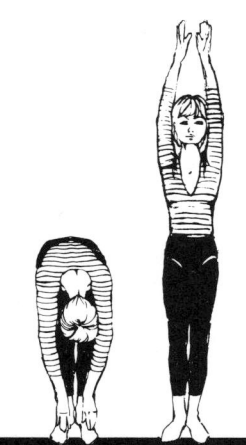

Feet very slightly apart. Bending knees, relax down over them towards the floor, arms held loosely in front. Slowly uncurl, stretching upwards with both arms towards the ceiling as you straighten up.

Chair exercises

Chair exercises can be very useful and I have given a series of exercises in Chapter 18, 'As young as you feel'. The body weight is taken by the chair so that it is less tiring to exercise the neck, shoulders, hands and feet than it would be if you were standing. Quite big movements can be done sitting down, and there is always the back of a heavy chair to hold on to if you want to do some leg swings to mobilise the hips. The main thing is to move and to keep moving.

Mini movements

If muscles are allowed to become slack there will be more strain on the joints which, coupled with wear and tear, are likely to become painful. Prevent this by making mini movements a habit. If you run through the exercises daily they will become automatic and any little stiffness or ache will disappear.

Hands, feet, shoulders and knees take a great deal of strain and need a little extra care to keep them easy and comfortable. They must never be allowed to get set, and therefore it is well worth the effort to keep them moving. The same applies to necks and backs. The daily walk will soon be a pleasure.

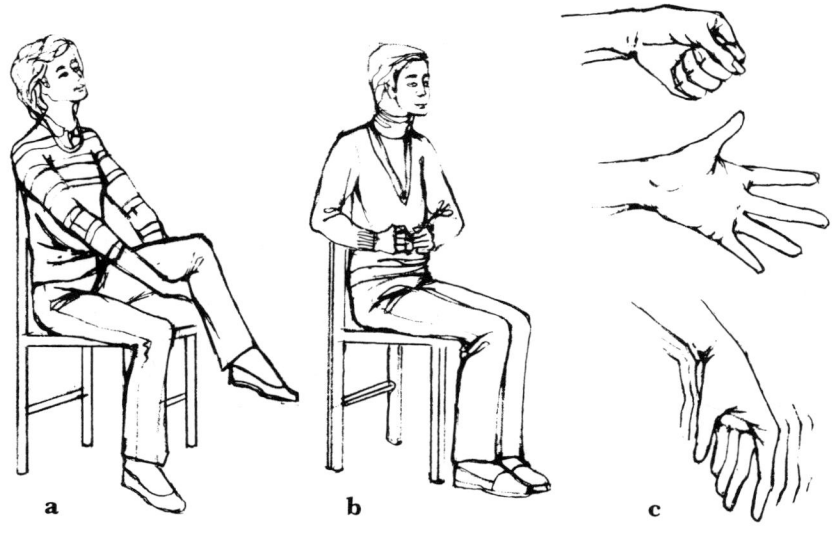

a Lift the knee and bend and stretch.

b Sit tall and well back in chair. With both hands on stomach muscles, pull in towards spine, and let go.

c Make a fist and stretch your fingers. Relax and shake them downwards from the wrist.

Water therapy

All through history we have heard about the healing merits of certain waters. Whether you consume it or sink into its comforting depths, water is wonderful. Considering how much water we all

For round shoulders

Pull a bath towel or scarf taut between both hands and raise high above head. Gently lower behind head while keeping head upright. Stretch towel again and bring down. Repeat several times.

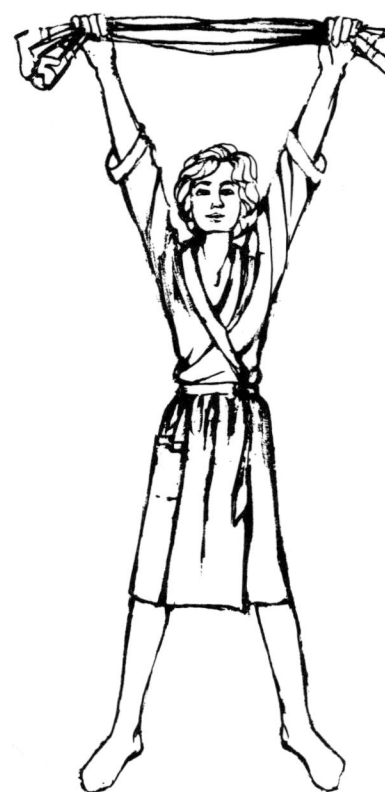

use, it is also very cheap and safe. Having reached a stage in our lives when time is not quite so important, the daily or even twice-daily bath comes into its own. It becomes almost a ritual; not too hot, not too cold, scented, bubbly or oily, according to taste.

The bath is even more beneficial if it is combined with a little exercise. We are in the mood, unrestrained by clothing and better able to stretch and bend for general mobility or to loosen up after a night's rest. According to the space available, movements can be large or small. A good upward stretch will ease out any temporary stiffness, and deep knee bending can be done holding on to the edge of the bath or washbasin. For round shoulders, catch hold of both ends of a bath towel, pull it taut and take it up and over your head, and keep it stretched at the back of your neck. Keep your head upright and strengthen your shoulders.

Foot exercises are easy to do in or under water. Try bending, stretching, and circling them from the ankles.

A good soak is relaxing, but not for too long. For further water therapy, swim in the sea whenever possible. If swimming must be in pools and your skin is dry, counteract the effect of the chlorine with hand or body lotion.

Drink up to six glasses of water each day; it is good for the complexion and the system. Do not be tempted to cut down on fluids in order to lose weight. Drinking plenty of water apparently has no connection with fluid retention, but dehydration on the other hand affects your looks and can lead to cramp.

Nutrition

If there is one subject that defies generalisation it is ageing. You simply cannot put people into categories today or tell at a glance how old they are – one person looks forty at sixty and another looks sixty at forty. I have noticed, however, that the younger-looking people nearly always watch what they eat. Although I think it is fair to say that a little extra weight can sometimes be kinder to the face and skin, I am sure that in the long run we need less food as we get older. I mean, of course, in quantity – not quality.

Nutrition is a fascinating subject and one well worth a little study. It is important for everyone to ensure that they eat enough protein each day as protein does not stay in the body and must be replenished daily. A deficiency will result in loss of energy and a decline in general health. Older people do not always bother to maintain a balanced diet and this can be a serious problem. Meat, fish, eggs and cheese are the basic types of protein foods, and a course of Vitamin B in tablet form is a good supplement if required.

Fresh fruit and lightly-cooked vegetables provide sufficient Vitamin C as a rule, but this could be pepped up in the winter. If you are feeling under the weather, a good boost is cod liver oil.

For any weakness in the bones (e.g. osteoporosis) which sometimes occurs in an elderly member of the family, calcium and phosphorus are strongly recommended. Milk, cheese, fish, spinach and dry beans are good sources of calcium, and eggs contain phosphorus. Calcium in some form helps if wakeful nights are a problem – and sugar, chocolate and cocoa should be avoided. Phosphorus is also good for the nerves.

I could write about nutrition for ever. By far the best thing to do is to discuss a suitable diet with your doctor.

Retirement reminders

1. If you cannot remember names of people and places, learn them all over again.

2. What happened recently is usually more entertaining than events of fifty years ago.

3. You learn more if you listen.

4. Stand tall and think tall.

5. There are usually more good days than bad.

6. Pay special attention to your feet. If they hurt, you are back in that chair.

7. If you don't know what to say when you leave your job, smile. Smile anyway.

8. Dance the old-fashioned way for hip mobility; it is dignified too.

9. Women – enjoy your friends. Men – keep yours.

10. Don't fuss. Be friendly. Feel fine.

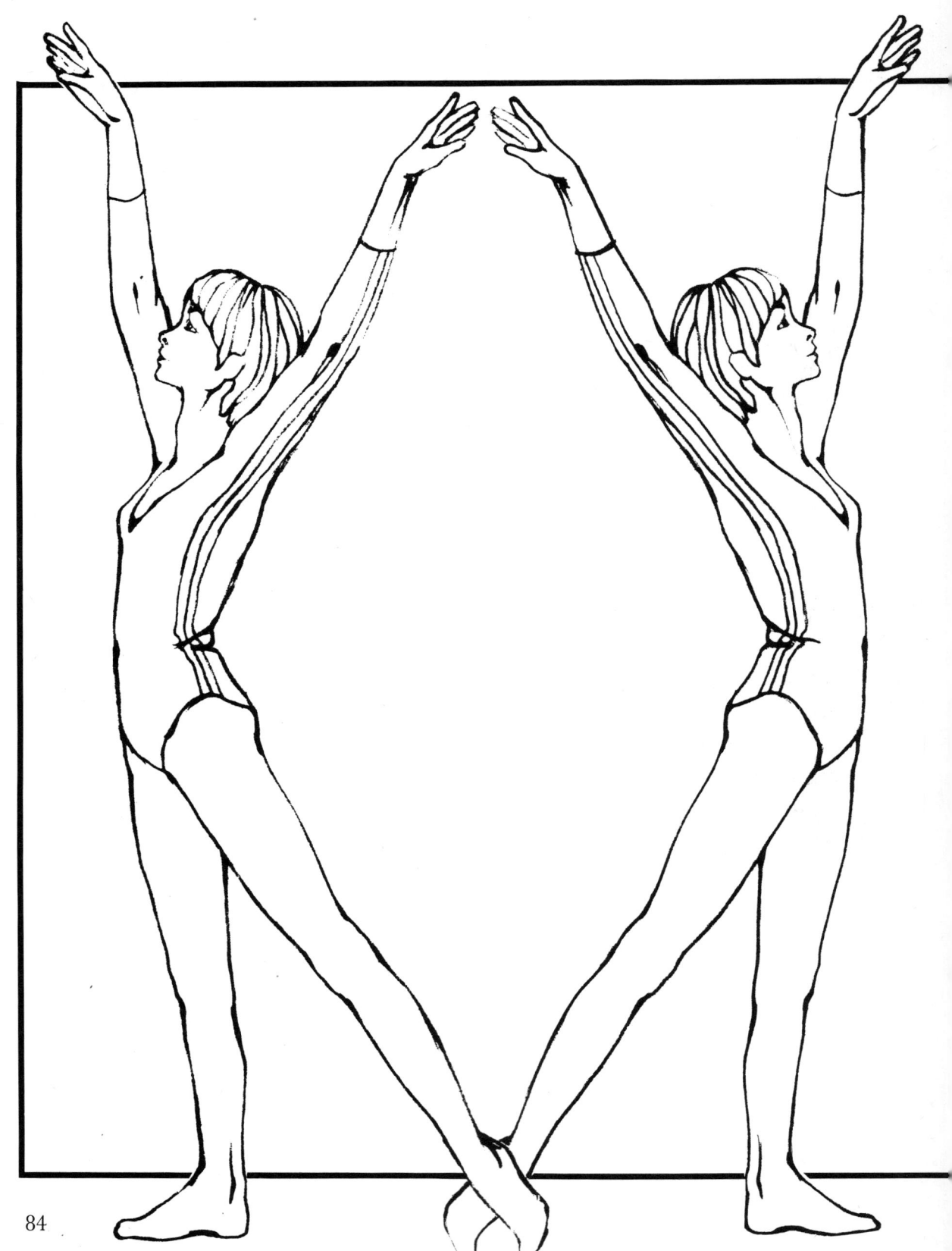

Chapter 8

Keeping fit at home

The aim of keep fit is to improve the health and looks and to promote a feeling of well-being. The emphasis is on personal enjoyment. Exercise for men and women. Introducing the exercises.
How to practise. Warm-ups. Where to start and what to wear. Basic rock and rhythmic walk exercises. Music to make you move. Terms of movement.

Keeping fit at home is very like joining a keep fit class. A class aims to improve the health and looks and to promote a feeling of well-being. The exercises stimulate circulation and strengthen and tone the muscles which support and control the figure. The emphasis at the class is on personal enjoyment. The desire to get up and exercise is not present in everyone, and class members must feel an overwhelming compulsion to join in. They must be given good reasons for doing so to justify the effort made, and they must feel for themselves the fascination of moving to music. Once persuaded by an irresistible rhythmic beat and the simplicity of the exercise, class members will try, and if they can follow easily the first time then they are extremely likely to continue. They feel younger and brighter, and have an amused sense of achievement at succeeding immediately with a new skill.

However, many people still look upon physical education as physical training and remember their own somewhat 'military' training at school. Because of this, at home or in a class it is necessary to start immediately to train a relaxed way of moving – a fluid and flowing way so that instead of isolated jerky exercise the whole body moves and brings more and more muscles into play. When the knees have lost their stiffness and relax automatically and when the change of weight from foot to foot becomes habit, then it is possible to move further and further in every direction and to cover as much space as possible.

In this way the body becomes completely mobile, supple and relaxed. Joints move freely and the figure 'fines' down as the constant stretching, bending and swinging helps to break down the deposits of fat, firms up the muscles and gives elasticity and flexibility to the whole.

As the circulation is stimulated, the fresh supply of blood to every part of the body brings with it a feeling of exhilaration. Regular practice helps to nourish the hair, skin and to improve the looks generally. Exercise strengthens heart and lungs, and this stimulates more vigorous breathing and a speeding up of the circulation throughout the body.

The modern dance steps and movements in the exercise routines help co-ordination, and the mind, too, is stimulated, leaving no room for personal problems. Afterwards these can be returned to refreshed.

Why women like keep fit

Every woman wants to be admired, however much she hides it! She feels that, given a chance, she could be as attractive as the next woman, and anything that can bring this goal in sight interests her. Her upbringing may prevent her from using artificial beauty aids or buying glamorous clothes, but if her common sense tells her that by following a simple routine she will achieve her object, then she will try. She already knows that she must not eat too much, that her face will become lined if she does not rest enough, that fresh air and the simplest skin care will help her to look young. Maybe her husband doesn't like dancing and she doesn't get the same amount of exercise as she was used to.

She is a potential candidate for a new hobby that will improve her looks and the way she feels. She is not interested enough, perhaps, to seek out a keep fit class, but bring it to her doorstep and she will join. If the movements are natural and vaguely familiar she will find that she is able to do them. She will see herself at the next party, walking into a strange room, poised and confident, standing tall, slim and graceful. She will go further. She will start to go for walks, to eat the right things, to put her feet up, to go to bed earlier, since she will realise that these things make all the difference in the world to the way she looks and feels. But she needs compulsion – it is easier to sit and dream.

Mainly for men

Men are also realising that if they want to stay young and active they must take some form of exercise. A sport or a routine of conditioning exercises is essential if muscles are not to become slack or joints set.

Most of the exercises in this book are suitable for both sexes – and men will certainly benefit from the whole book. The exercise routine in Chapter 14 is especially designed for strength, endurance and mobility. The exercises are not very strenuous as they stand, but repetition will make them so. Care should be taken while performing floor exercises and if abdominal muscles have

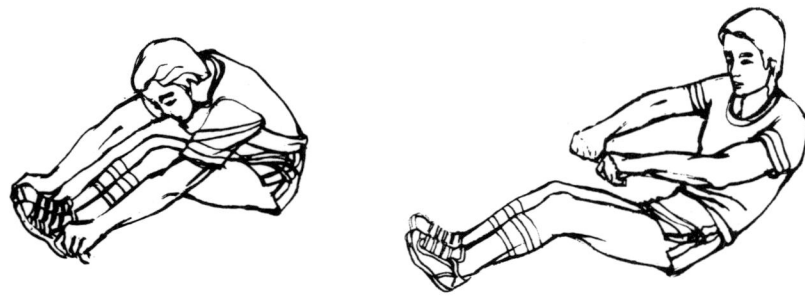

Rowing exercise

become slack then only a few repeats should be included at first. Back and stomach muscles work together and both can give trouble if strained.

A good test for slack muscles is to lie flat on the floor and sit up without help from the hands. If this is easy, there should be no flabbiness of the muscles. Another test is to sit on the floor and row – moving forward and back as if rowing a boat. If you can hold the halfway back position, then the muscles are pretty firm. Running on the spot for a short time also gives an idea of general condition.

The exercises

The exercise sequences and routines are arranged in chapters, and each individual exercise has a title. The exercises are straightforward, self-explanatory and easy to follow. The drawings show how each movement should look and clear instructions are given to describe each step. Many of the stretching and bending movements are part of our daily lives; the training simply ensures that we move in the right way with an economy of effort.

The exercises have been arranged to prevent anyone from becoming unduly tired by using the same group of muscles for too long. You will notice that the muscle groups are constantly changed during a routine. If we start with an arm and shoulder movement, we change to a leg exercise so that the first group of muscles rests. This may be followed by a floor exercise for the abdominal muscles, where the body weight is taken by the floor. In this way we finish the session not exhausted, but refreshed. It is therefore very important to practise a routine in the order given. In addition to the changing of muscle groups you may want to add a break. Breaks are not always necessary, but after a strong exercise you may find that a swing, hand, foot or dance movement can be relaxing and give variety to the sequence. Some of the exercise sequences finish in this manner.

The chapters contain general stretching exercises to encourage good posture and to teach all members of the family how to stand, sit and walk tall. There are exercises to fine down the figure, emphasising the 'lift' of the chest which allows the body to fall into line. In all the routines there are exercises to promote a relaxed way of moving from the feet upwards, obtained through the change of weight from foot to foot and easy knees. This is the basis of modern keep fit. Sequences encourage movement in every direction for uplift, waistline and stomach muscles. The accent is always on easy knees in order for the practitioner to move further to his or her fullest capacity.

While new to the exercises, I suggest supported positions for hip mobility and deep knee bending. It is advisable to hold on to the back of a chair while learning to swing, circle and lift alternate legs. These leg exercises are important to encourage movement in every direction, to loosen the hip joints and to emphasise relaxation in the knees and the use of weight during leg swings.

Certain small mobility movements are easier to do sitting in a chair. These include head turning and circling to mobilise muscles of the neck and to firm the line of the chin, and rotation and shrugging of shoulders for good posture. Shoulder shrugging relaxes tension and breaks down any fatty deposits at the back of the neck (which can be the start of a 'dowagers hump'). Mobility movements for upper arms, hands and wrists, knees, ankles and feet prevent gradual and sometimes unnoticed slowing down of movement in unused muscles and joints.

Floor exercises mean that the body weight is supported by the floor. The exercises are fairly strong and vigorous in order to fine down the figure and strengthen the muscles of the back, abdomen, hips and thighs.

The dance routines are suitable for everyone. They include special fencing-type lunging movements, stretching and relaxing and spinal curl exercises to increase balance and poise.

Progressive exercise

In Chapters 9 to 13 the exercises are progressive, so it is important to start at the beginning and work up to the more advanced movements in Chapter 15. Chapter 14 contains exercises which are particularly suitable for men, but can be followed by women too. For the newcomer, it is essential to start slowly and to condition the body gradually. Experienced movers will probably prefer to use the routines how and when they choose.

Chapters 16 to 18 are in a different category. 'Morning Choice', Chapter 16, is a two-minute routine and it should be practised straight away. 'Muscular relaxation', Chapter 17, teaches the recognition of tension, and 'As young as you feel', Chapter 18, is for those who prefer to sit.

How to practise

You will need space in which to move, so make sure that there is no furniture in your immediate vicinity. Push back the chairs and tables and see that the carpet is clear and that there are no mats around which could trip you up. This may sound very elementary advice, but if you make your home your gymnasium such matters as space and safety are very important.

Clothing will depend on the time of day you exercise and whether you choose to practise in the bedroom, bathroom or sitting room. If you are at home, then trousers and a loose top are ideal. Leotards and track suits are fine for class wear. Many people prefer to practise in bare feet but I think that soft slippers are safer, provided they fit properly. You should *never* exercise in flip flops.

Have a record or cassette player handy; music makes you move.

Warm-up

Now for the warm-up. This is essential. However short of time you are, never start an exercise routine from cold – even running through 'Morning Choice' will do as a warm-up.

Check your posture first. Stand with your back to a clear piece of wall and stretch up with one arm at a time. Each arm should lie flat on the wall close to your head as in the posture test in Chapter 1. Now devise your own warm-up. Reach and clap up and down and to either wall, run, dance or do anything that will get you going.

Start with the first three exercises in Chapter 9. Get those three right first before you tackle the rest of the routine and move on to later chapters.

Daily practice

As you proceed day by day you will find that you can move more easily and you may be tempted to go on and on. Ultimately, you can work for an hour if you feel like it, but for the first week or two just ten minutes a day is enough. You can gradually build up to twenty, and so on. If you stiffen up you will not feel like starting again, so it is far better at the end of your session to go out and walk for ten minutes to loosen up.

Never practise immediately after a meal or too late at night. Just yawn and stretch a few times to relax. On rising your 'Morning Choice' routine is best. Arrange your main practice session for later in the day.

If you were attending a fashionable dance centre, the walls would be covered with mirrors so that you would be able to check every movement you made. This would help considerably in improving your performance. Observation is of the greatest value in the early stages of practice, and even more so if your aim is to become a keep fit leader or teacher.

Most people have a long mirror somewhere in the house and it is well worth while watching yourself move, otherwise it could feel as if your arm were really stretching upwards, perfectly straight, but if you looked in the mirror you would see that it was bending at the elbow. The arm could be away from the side of your head instead of close to it, as in the diagrams, so watch yourself more. See exactly what is happening and correct any fault early on. Any tendency to round shoulders can also be seen in a mirror. It is not easy to *feel* that you are standing perfectly straight, especially when you are tired. I know of someone who habitually carries his left shoulder higher than his right, and simply does not believe it until he looks in the mirror.

When exercising on the floor a mirror is not such a help, but a session with an enthusiastic keep fit friend can help to correct any faults, and is usually great fun.

Basic rock

There is one movement I would like you to learn now, and this is the Basic Rock. The Basic Rock is the change of weight from foot to foot which forms the basis of many exercises. It is 'feet wide apart and stand easy' and you will need to know how to do it.

Relax your knees and let yourself sway gently from foot to foot – take your weight over but remain upright yourself. The feet, ankles and knees should do all the work. It is almost as if you were standing on the deck of a ship and trying to keep your balance.

Why do we need this movement? The answer is simply because it allows you to move more. You can stretch further to the right if you rock right – try it! If we always stood with feet rigidly together the exercises would become stale. Of course, with a deep knee

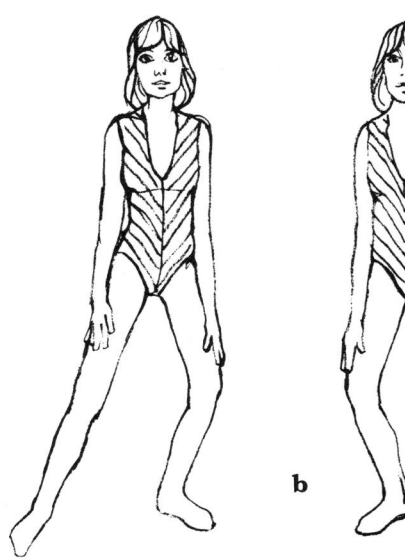

a   b

Basic rock
a Feet wide apart, relax knees and take weight over to left foot.
b 'Rock' your weight back to right foot – knees bending slightly as weight goes across, arms relaxed at sides.

91

bend, feet are usually together, but when we must really move our whole body, we need to rely on the Basic Rock.

Rhythmic walk

If you were to join a keep fit class you would probably find that a good deal of floor space is covered between the movements. Choreography is important, particularly if demonstrations are planned, and class members are trained to move from place to place. In this way, attractive patterns can be formed which are a pleasure to watch.

In keep fit, a rhythmic walk or run is often used to change the pattern. This is an exercise in itself, and whether the walking is done rhythmically in class or as a leisure activity, the procedure is much the same. These points should be kept in mind at first, then forgotten so that the walk is entirely natural.

1. The feet should be kept as parallel as possible, neither turned out nor in.

2. The head should be held high, completely in line with the spine, with eyes level.

3. Heels should touch the ground lightly, with the weight rolling on to the ball of the foot.

4. Knees should be loose, never stiff.

5. Hip joints should be kept free with leg exercises, allowing a reasonable step forward but not a stride.

6. Momentum is gained by pushing off with the back foot, arms swinging freely.

7. Balance and relaxation will ensure a good carriage. There should be no rigidity.

8. Shoulders should be relaxed and down, never high and tense.

9. A feeling of 'lift' from the chest should pervade the whole body.

Rhythmic running is an extension of walking, but on the ball of the foot – arms relaxed at sides.

Music to make you move

Music certainly makes you want to move. But to move to your fullest capacity you need time. Sometimes very fast music can tie you down and prohibit movement as you endeavour to stay on the beat. It is generally more helpful to use a variety of tempos, and in many cases the movement should control the music. For instance, to extend your range of movement allow plenty of time by using a slow waltz or four: four time to exercise to.

At home it is important to vary the pace of the exercises as much as possible. When you choose your music get some contrast into your session if you can by following a slow tempo for a big movement with a quick tempo for a warm-up or break. For small movements, go for something lively with a beat. You do not have to move on every beat of the bar; you can take a couple of bars to stretch and come back to the beat for a shoulder shrug. When setting simple vigorous movements to pop music, try counting eight. There may be odd bars, and the music will run on, but at least you will know where you are. You can count eight four times to cover one step or movement; change the step for the next four eights, and so on, until you have a routine. Get to know your music thoroughly and adapt accordingly. There are endless ways to use your music, and it is fun to experiment as long as the music helps the movement and does not hinder it.

Chapters 9, 10, 11, 12 and 18 have been recorded under the overall titles of the routines. (See Chapter 20.) Here the music has been specially composed to give the utmost support to the exercises. For the other sequences I have suggested tempos. There is so much taped music available that it should not be difficult to set the movements to suitable tunes, whether old favourites or with a modern beat.

There is no doubt that using appropriate music makes all the difference and encourages that feeling of tremendous vitality which exercise brings, even if you are feeling a little off-colour and not a bit like exercising.

Terms of movement

Beat: To slap with flat of hand on or across knees and thighs, as in Tyrolean dancing.

Bend: If bending forwards and down, the knees must bend.

Break: Any kind of step or small movement in between strong exercises; to break any tension.

Circle: Used for wrists, hands, ankles, knees, head, shoulders and whole body.

Dig: A movement with the ball of the foot; often used instead of step and close (i.e. when weight is kept on standing foot and not transferred so that the other foot is ready to use).

Drop down: To flop like a rag doll over knees.

Finger snap: With thumb and third finger, used in Spanish type movement or jazz.

Fling: A quick relaxed stretch of the arm.

Fold: To cross the arms.

Kick: A quick leg lift from the hips.

Knee bounce: Easy bending of the knees more than once.

Lift: A lift of the chest, felt throughout the body.

Pull: With a fist, as if pulling on a rope.

Punch: With a fist, bend and then stretch arm.

Push: A stretching movement, bending the elbow or knee first.

Reach out: To stretch as far as possible.

Relax: To let go completely.

Rock: To change weight from foot to foot.

Stretch: To extend any part of the body to its greatest capacity.

Support: In the home, hold on to a chair back or piece of heavy furniture to aid balance for a leg exercise; in class, hold hands with a partner.

Sweep: A wide movement of arm and hand overhead from right to left, or left to right.

Swing: A rhythmic movement of arm or leg, side to side, or forward and back; if a swing with arms, the body follows through.

Turn: Step to right side with right foot, across with left foot, turning to right, step right, facing front.

Twist: Used for waistline; feet wide apart and knees relaxed to allow upper part of body to turn to side or back.

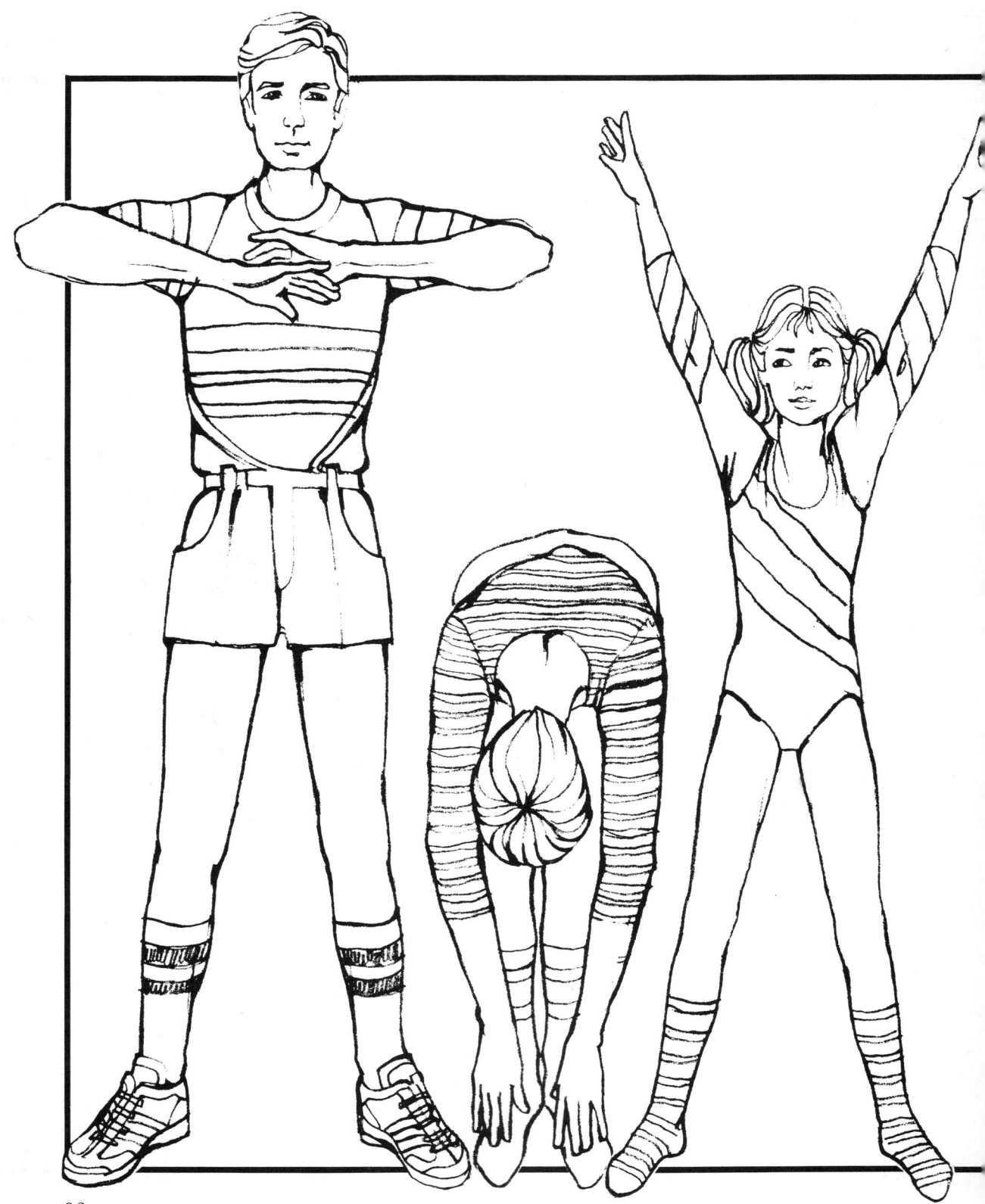

Chapter 9

Family keep-fit

An exercise routine for all members of the family

From the very beginning of this routine you will see that the accent is on good posture. It is very important to stand tall, and the first exercise encourages this. The leg swings which follow need strong support, and it is important to hold on to something which is very firm and at the correct height.

When lying on the floor for the abdominal exercises, relax the back as much as possible – relax into the floor, leaving no space between the floor and the small of the back. Should it be hard at first to lift, bend and stretch both legs together, try one at a time, as shown.

For a break in the floor exercises, lie still and pull hard on the stomach muscles. Pull them in towards the spine, hold, and let go. This is an excellent habit to acquire as it quickly strengthens the muscles. The exercise can be done sitting or standing as well.

When lunging forward, preferably right or left of centre as shown in exercise 8, the weight should be evenly distributed between both feet – the front foot in line with the leg, the back foot turned out. This fencing type movement improves posture and is particularly suitable for men.

For recorded music, see Chapter 20.

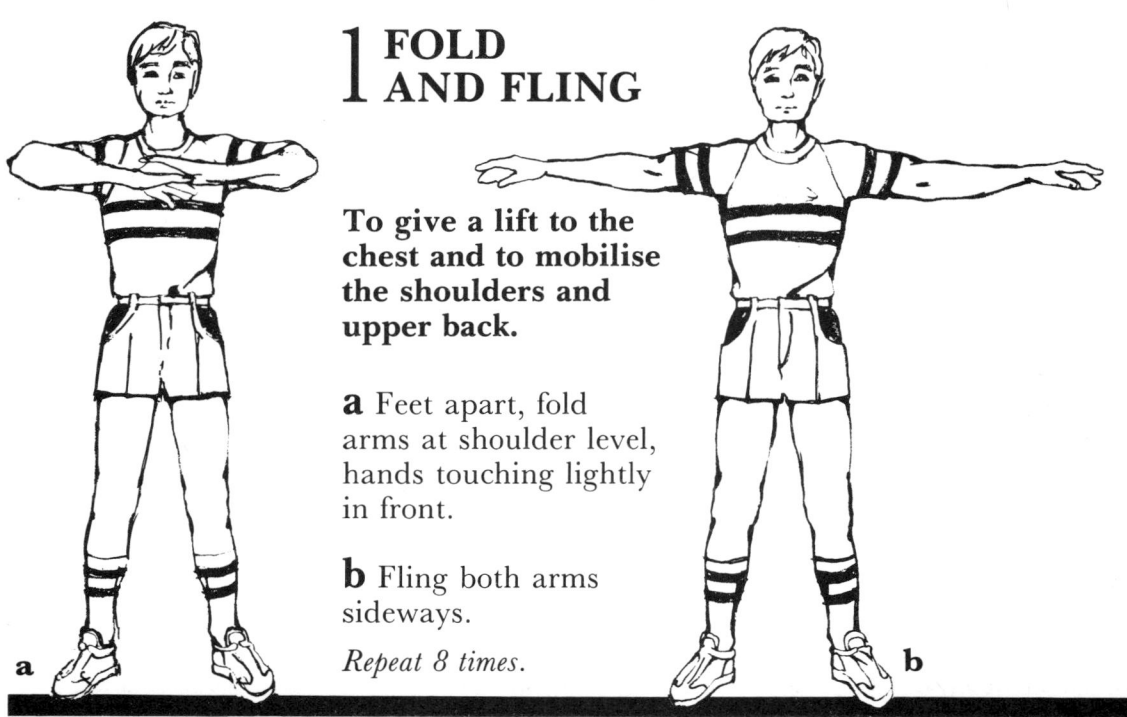

1 FOLD AND FLING

To give a lift to the chest and to mobilise the shoulders and upper back.

a Feet apart, fold arms at shoulder level, hands touching lightly in front.

b Fling both arms sideways.

Repeat 8 times.

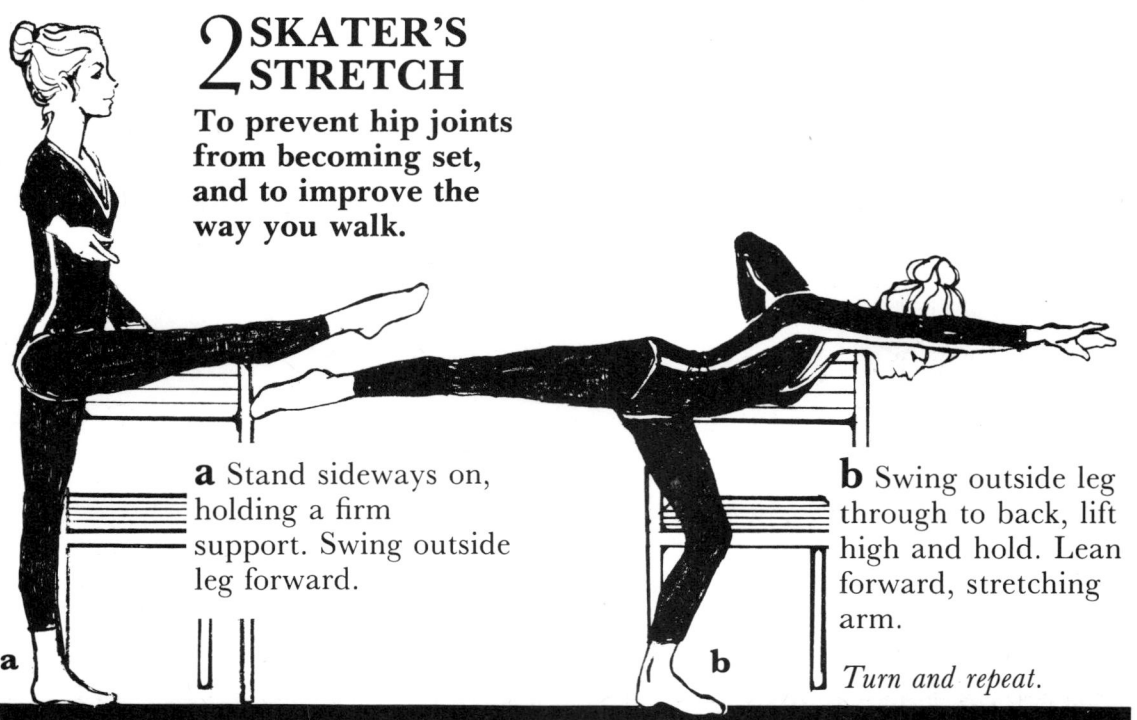

2 SKATER'S STRETCH

To prevent hip joints from becoming set, and to improve the way you walk.

a Stand sideways on, holding a firm support. Swing outside leg forward.

b Swing outside leg through to back, lift high and hold. Lean forward, stretching arm.

Turn and repeat.

3 CLAP HIGH, CLAP LOW

A full body stretch and relaxed drop to the floor to give elasticity to the figure.

a Reach high and clap 4 times overhead.

b Bend knees, relax down, and clap 4 times.

Change to clapping twice up and twice down, then once.

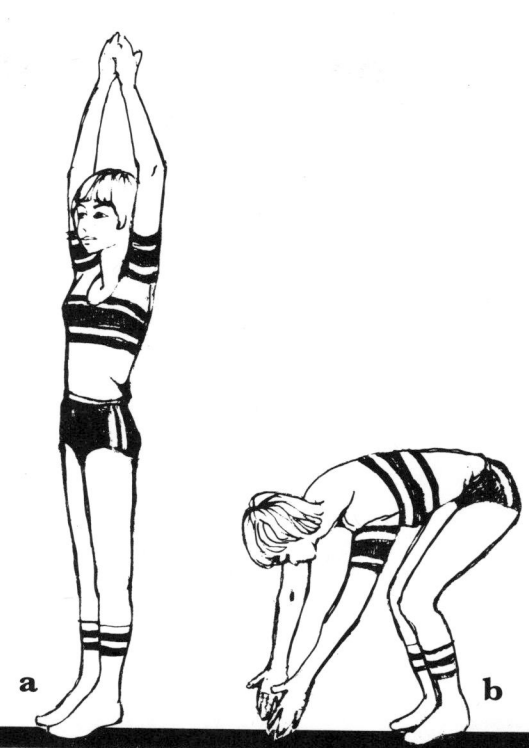

4 HEEL TOUCH

To train the knees to bend easily, and to tighten the seat muscles.

a Step on to right foot, bend left knee and raise foot to touch left hand. Lift opposite arm to aid balance.

b Drop left foot, raise right and touch it.

Repeat.

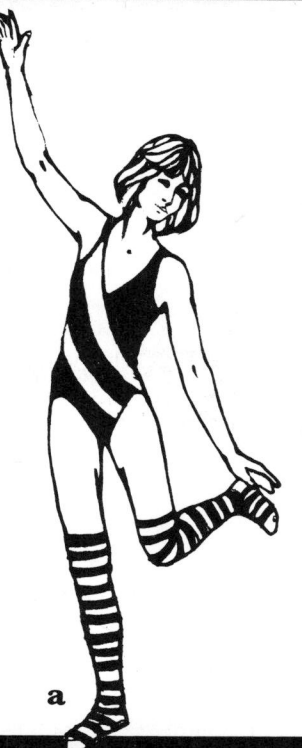
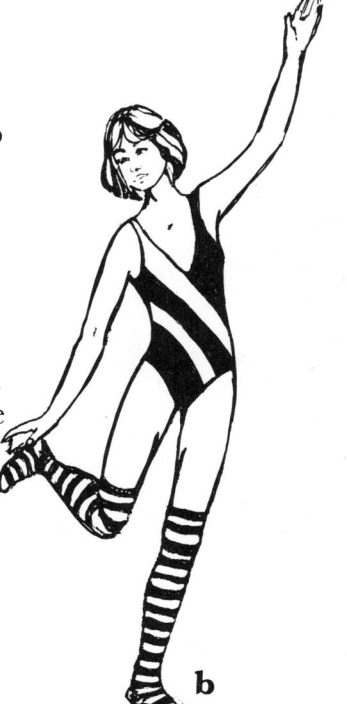

5 CAN CAN KICK

To strengthen lower abdominal muscles.

a Lie with left knee bent and right leg straight.

b Kick high 3 times with straight leg.

Change legs – bend right, straighten left and repeat.

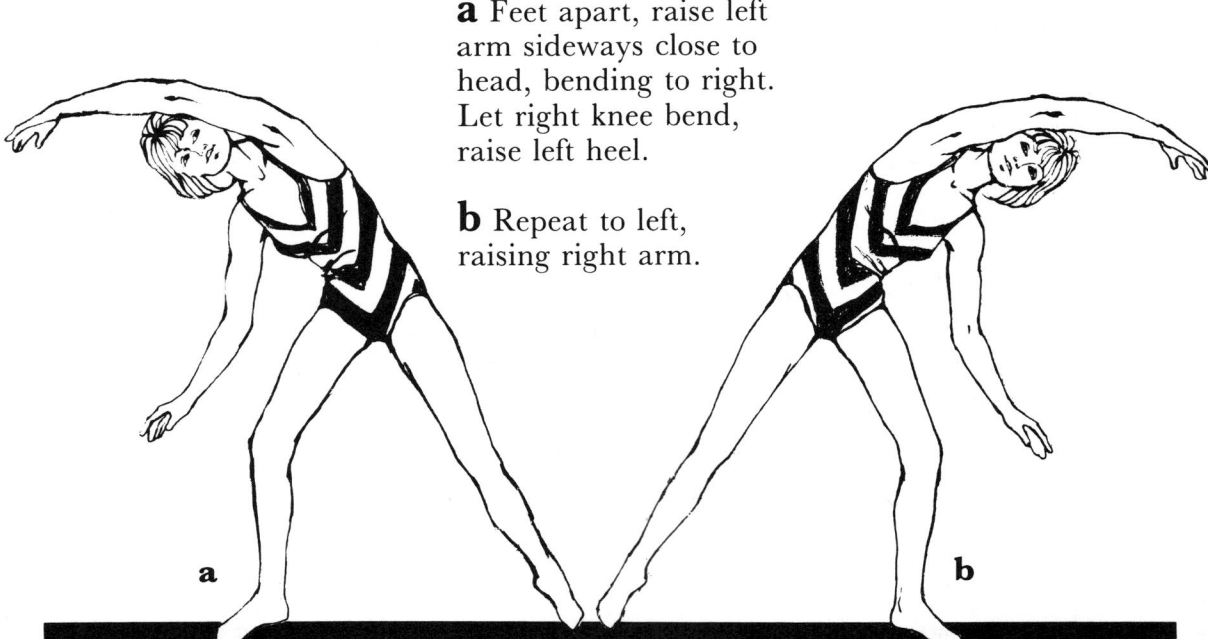

6 SIDE STRETCH

To firm a flabby waistline.

a Feet apart, raise left arm sideways close to head, bending to right. Let right knee bend, raise left heel.

b Repeat to left, raising right arm.

c Bend both knees towards chest.

d Stretch legs towards ceiling, bend and lower to floor.

Repeat c and d.

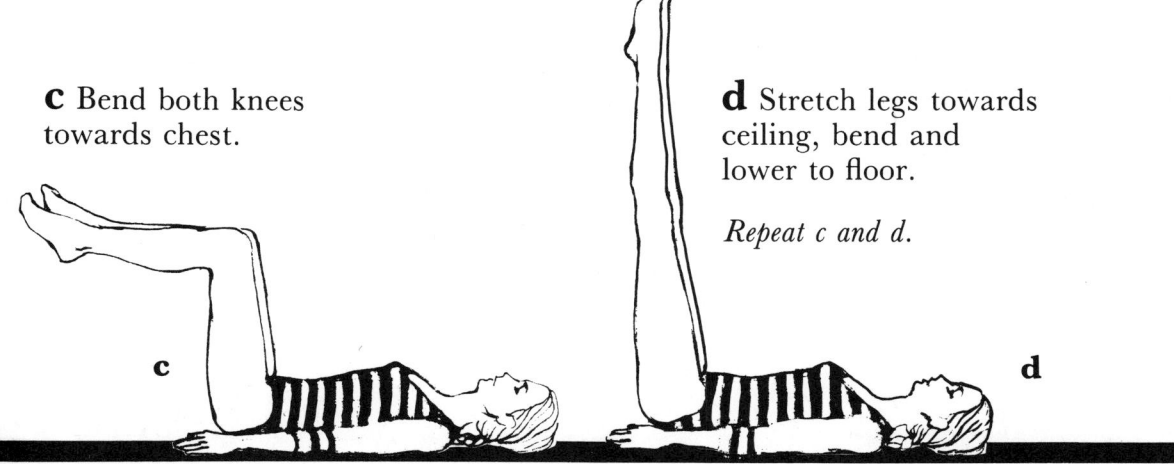

7 HIP WALK

A well-tried exercise to mobilise hips and reduce seat.

a Walk forward on seat, lifting alternate hips and arms.

b Walk back the same way.

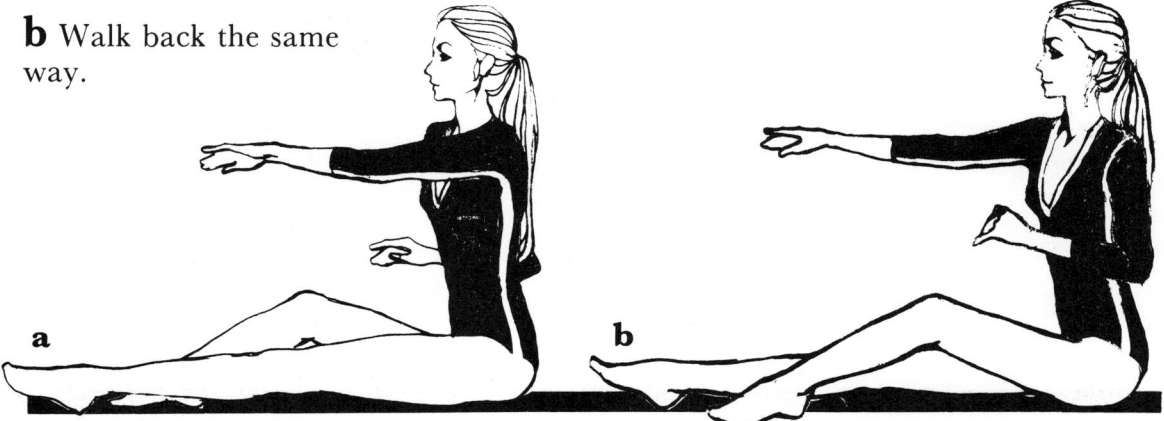

88 LUNGE FOR LINE

A classic fencing-type movement to improve posture.

a Raise arms sideways to V position while taking a big step forward with right foot. Right knee bends as left leg straightens.

b Drop arms and return, closing right foot to left.

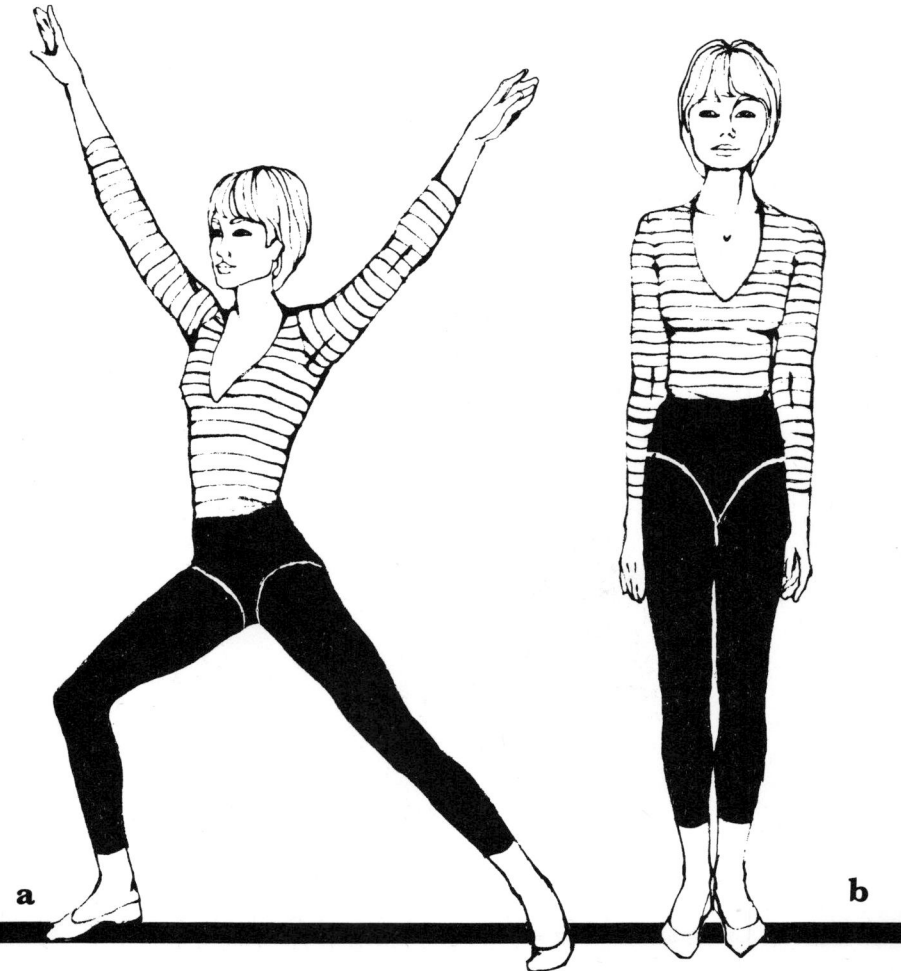

c Repeat with left foot.

d Return, closing left foot to right.

e Relax and flop over bent knees towards floor. Pull up – stand tall.

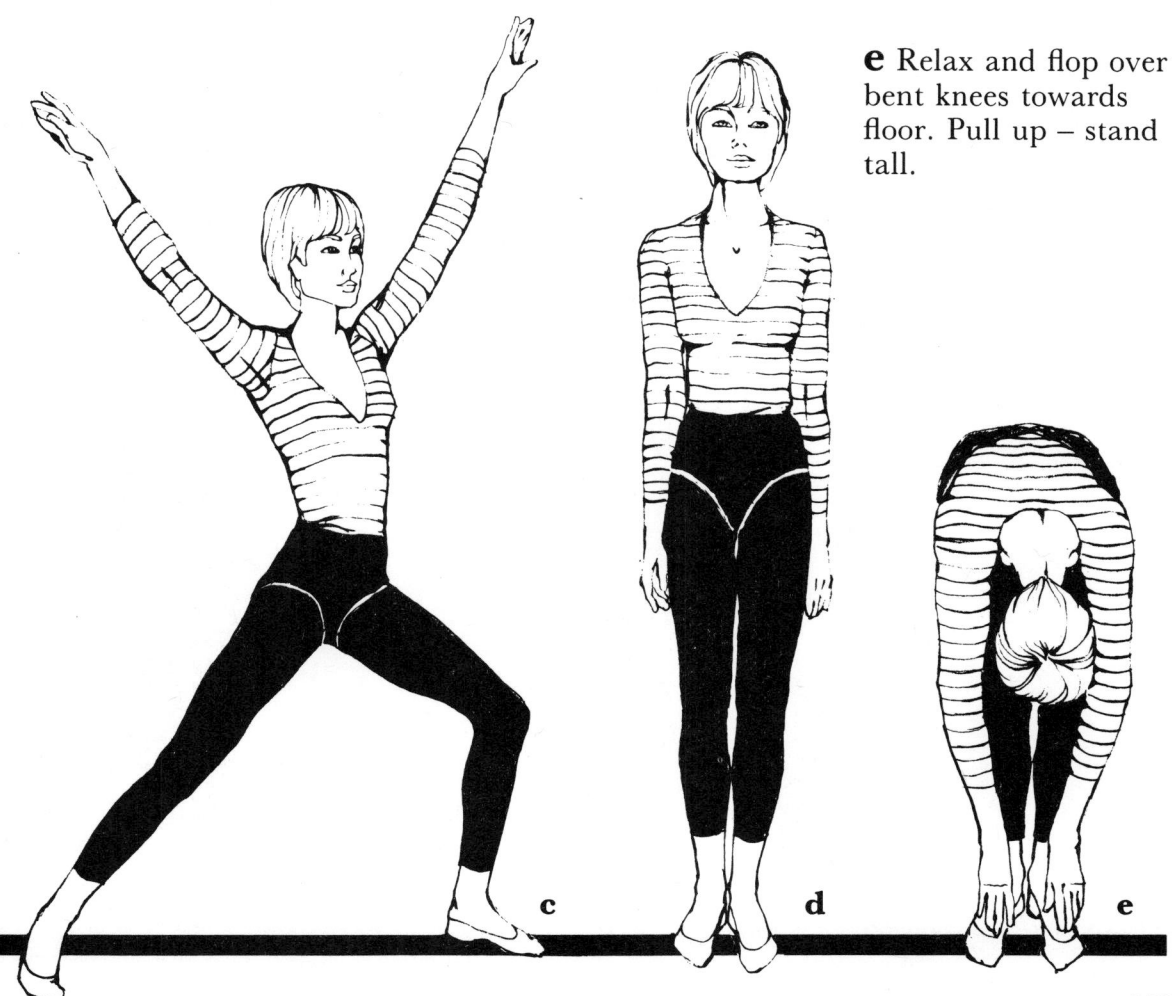

c d e

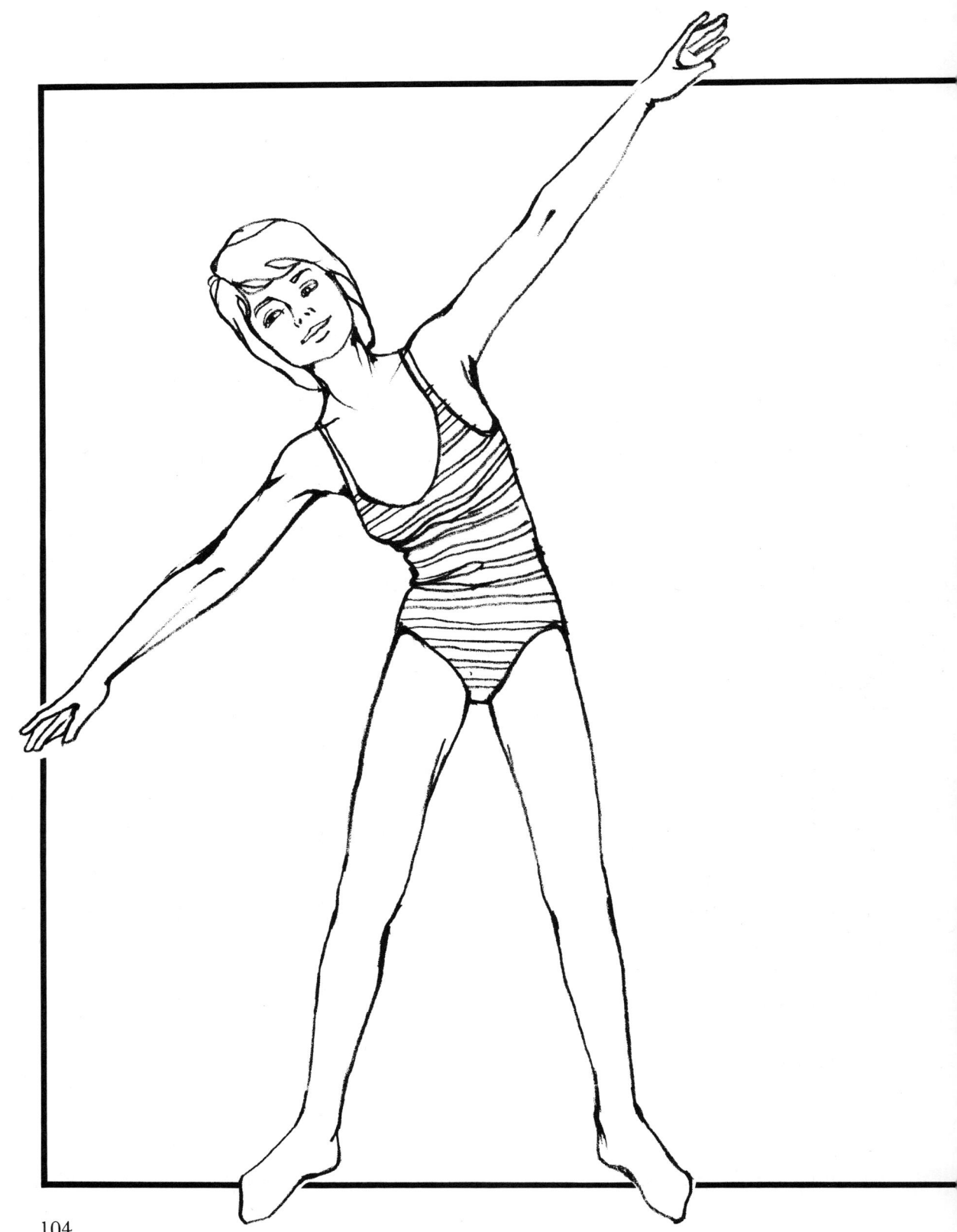

Chapter 10

Enjoy your slimming

A special sequence to trim the figure

Coupled with a sensible diet, these exercises will help you to lose weight. They will train the supporting muscles and correct any faults in posture which might have been caused by overweight. The routine will encourage a feeling of renewed energy and vitality, and all the exercises should be practised regularly with a sense of enjoyment.

The emphasis is on stretching and bending, and attention is concentrated on muscle groups in those areas where overweight shows first. This sequence should form part of your slimming programme at the first sign of any thickening of the body.

You will see from the drawings that more than half of the exercises are concerned with strengthening the stomach and thigh muscles. In exercise 6, both legs are lifted straight up from the floor at the same time. If this requires a great deal of effort, lift one leg at a time. Stomach and thighs will still benefit. Remember that a short work-out every day is always better than a long session once a week.

If music is required, see Chapter 20.

Enjoy your slimming

1 THE LADDER

To avoid a thickening waistline and to ease an aching back.

a Raise right arm sideways close to head, stretch high.

b Raise left arm up sideways, stretching higher.

Keep stretching upwards – higher and higher – with each arm alternately.

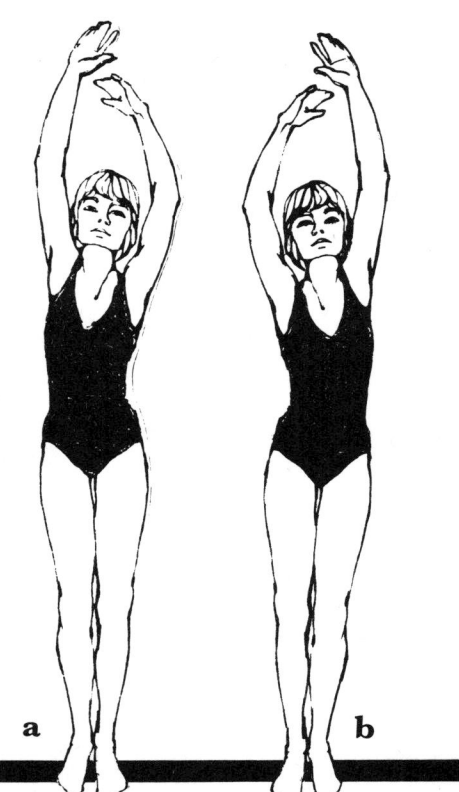

a   b

2 KNEE CLASP

A natural movement for stomach muscles, and preparation for stronger exercises.

Lie completely flat, or with feet higher than head. Pull alternate knees up close to chest, stretch, and put down.

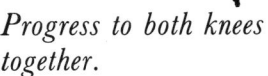

Progress to both knees together.

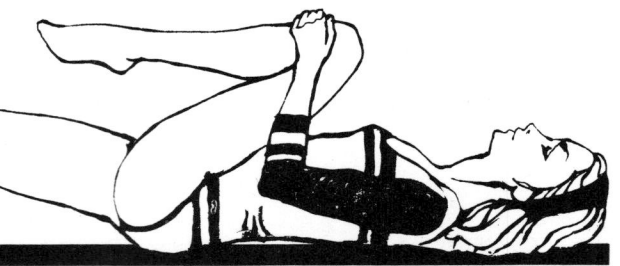

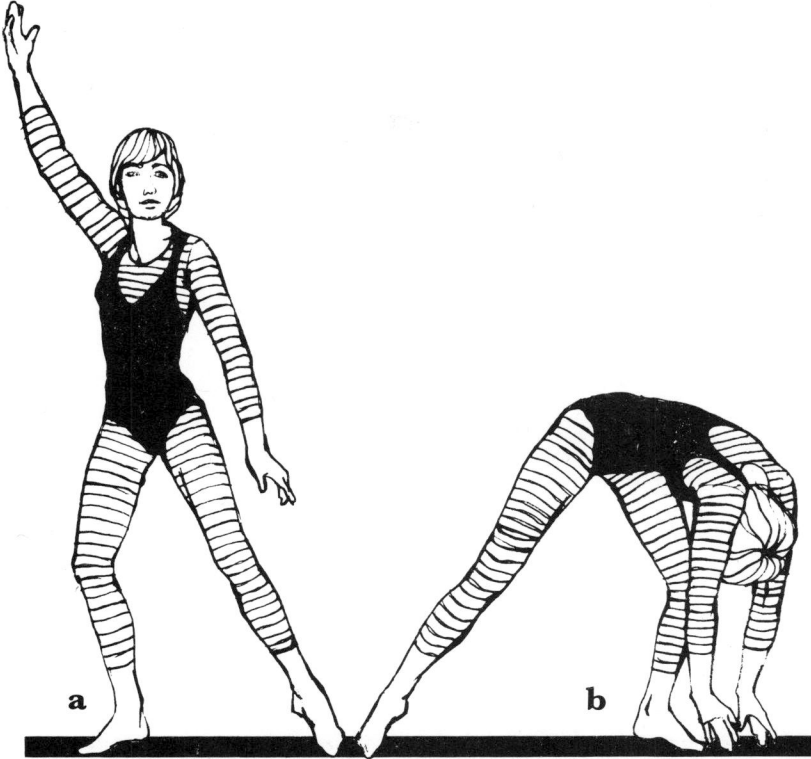

3 CIRCLE TOUCH TOE

A two-directional exercise to strengthen muscles above and below the waistline.

a Circle right arm forward, up, back and down, 4 times.

b Swing right arm forward and down to touch left toe, straighten up.

Repeat with left arm.

4 ROLL AND REACH

To reduce hips and seat.

a Sit on the floor, hands at either side.

b Roll on to left hip and hand, raising right arm to reach across to touch floor beyond.

Repeat to other side.

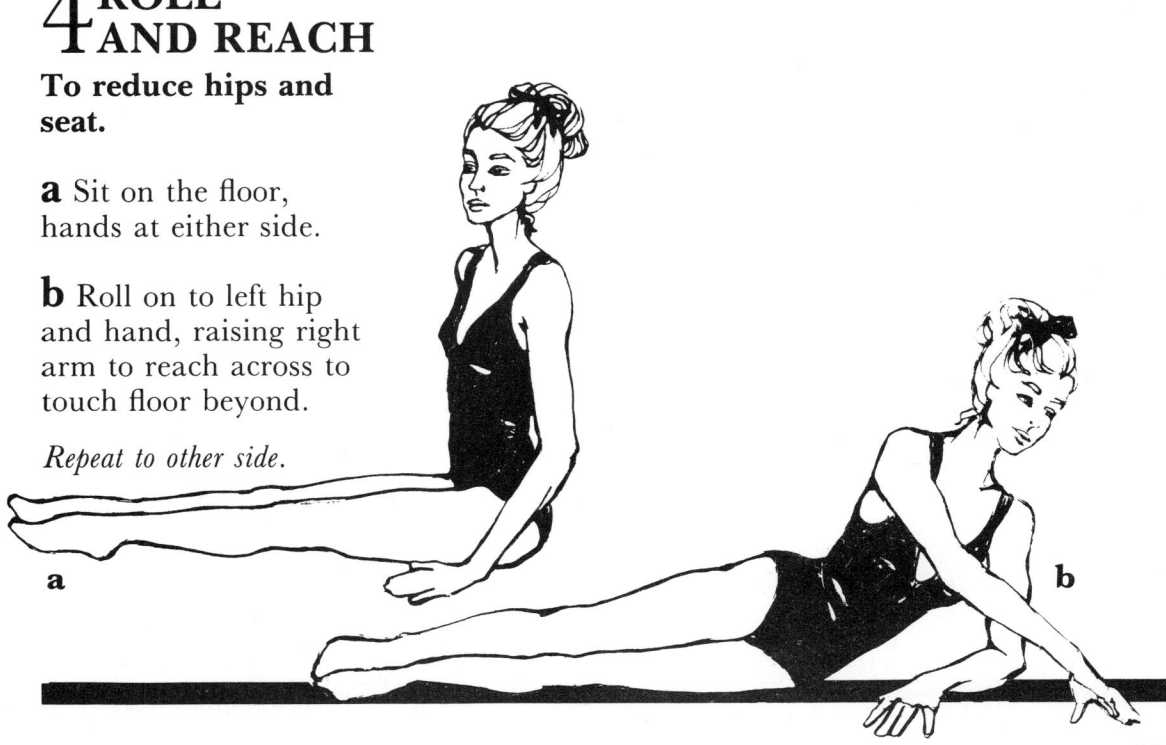

107

5 THE WINDMILL

A waistline winner.

a With feet apart and arms outstretched at shoulder level, bend sideways to right.

b Change direction and bend to left.

Gradually increase movements.

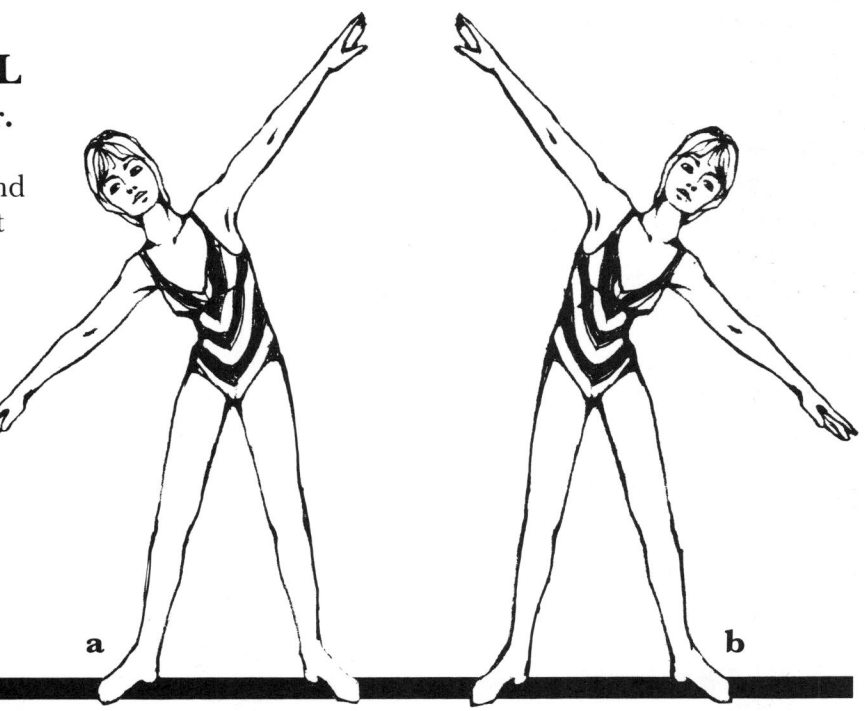

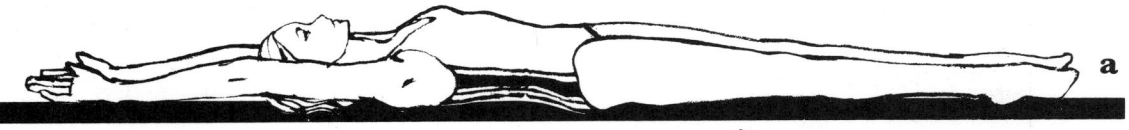

6 HAIRPIN BEND

To reduce abdomen and to tighten thigh muscles.

a Lie flat on floor. Stretch both arms up and behind head, keep legs straight.

b Raise arms and legs at the same time to touch at ankles or knees. Hold and lower both to floor, as at start.

Repeat.

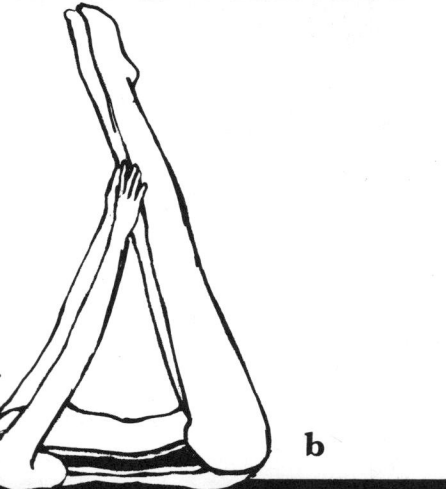

7 ROLLING PIN ROLL

A comprehensive exercise to fine down the figure and to strengthen the back and stomach muscles.

a With feet together, drop forward and down over knees.

b With imaginary rolling pin held close, roll it up your body, bending elbows.

c Roll yourself out completely, stretch high.

Repeat from this position.

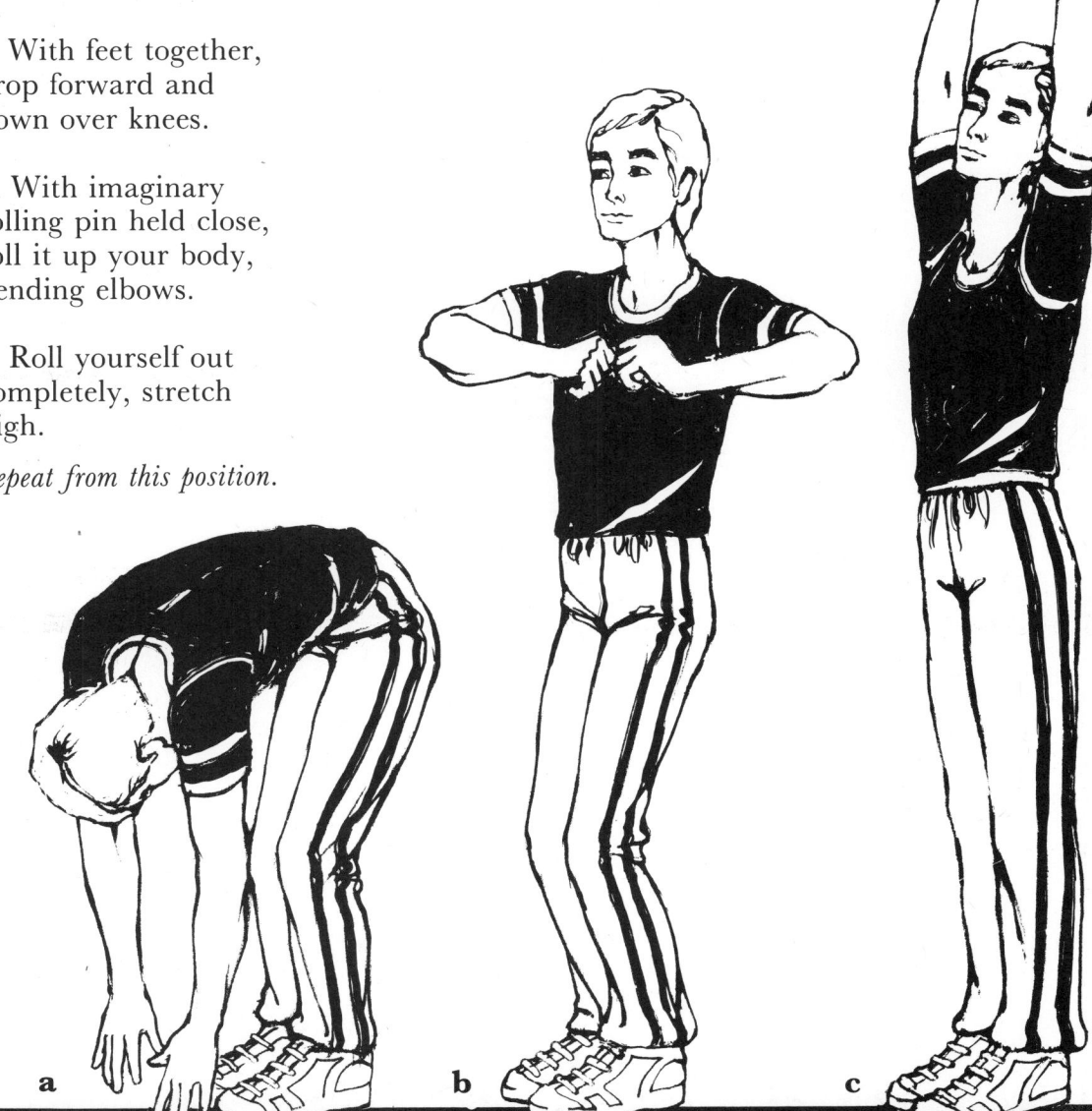

a   b   c

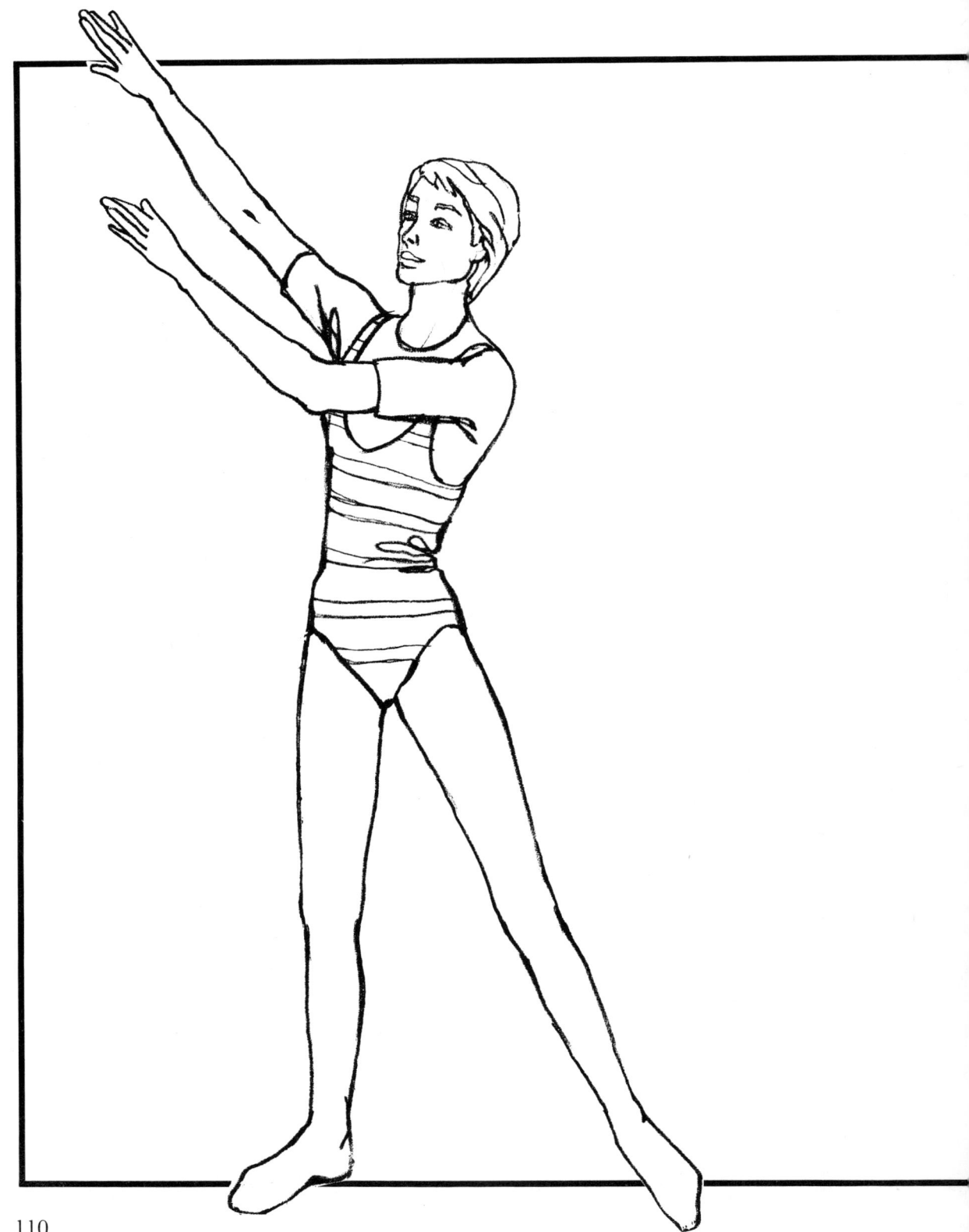

Chapter 11

Slim
to rhythm

Exercises for the young and the energetic

For these exercises I have in mind those who prefer a quicker pace and welcome a more vigorous routine. The movements are not complicated, and they can, of course, be taken more slowly if required.

Rhythm is very important for this sequence, and modern rhythm – tango or a disco beat – will suit most of the exercises, but it is best to swing to waltz time. You will notice that most of the movements depend on easy knees for their pace and general performance. Before you start, it would be wise to limber up with a few simple knee bends if your knees are inclined to be stiff.

I hope that you will enjoy these exercises. Do them with zest; they can be very exhilarating and should leave you with a sense of balance and poise.

For records and tapes, see Chapter 20.

1 KNOCK HIGH KNOCK LOW

A body line-up to straighten shoulders.

a Take arms up sideways, knock fists overhead, twice.

b Bring arms down and knock fists twice behind back.

Repeat. Shrug shoulders to relax arms.

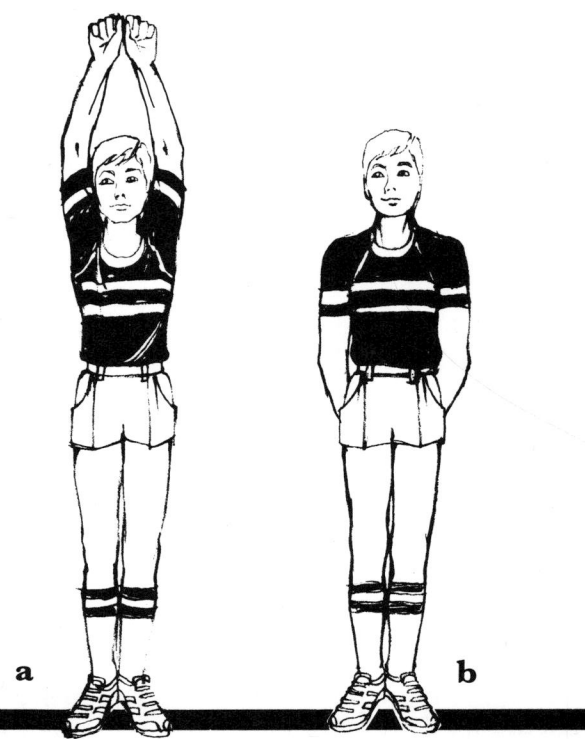

2 FLOOR STRETCH

For a leaner look.

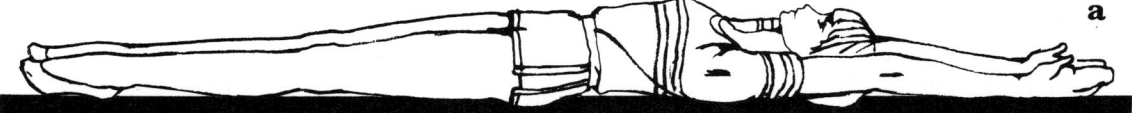

a Lie flat on the floor with both arms stretched behind the head.

b Bend knees, clasp and pull close to chest. Pull and pull.

Stretch legs and arms as before, and repeat.

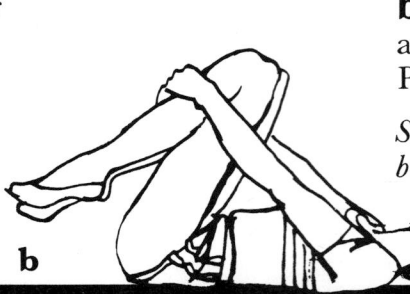

3 SWINGTIME (1) SWING HIGH

To give a lift to the figure, with the accent on waistline.

a With feet wide apart, swing both arms high to right.

b Repeat to left. Keep arms relaxed – no tension.

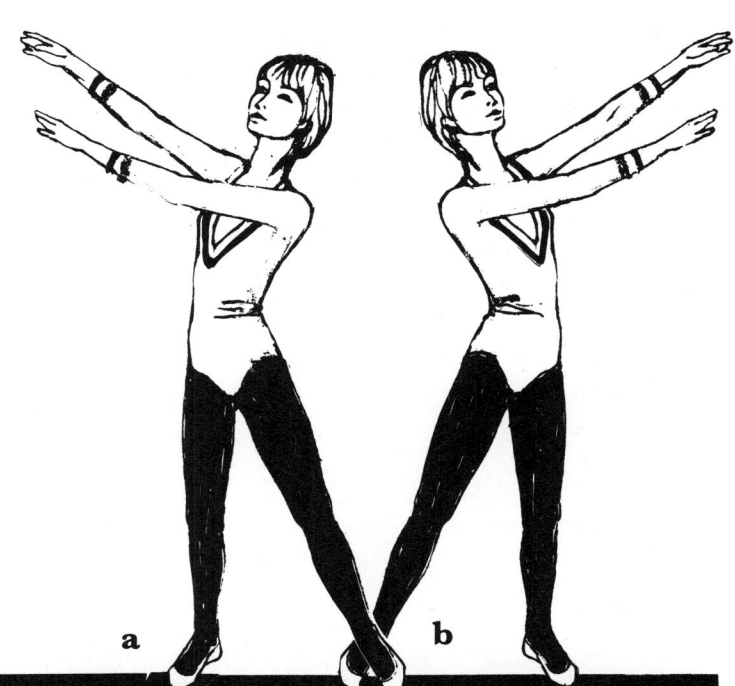

4 SWINGTIME (2) SWING LOW

To strengthen stomach muscles.

a Relax over bent knees, swinging to right, just above floor.

b Head well down, swing to left.

Repeat Swing High and Swing Low.

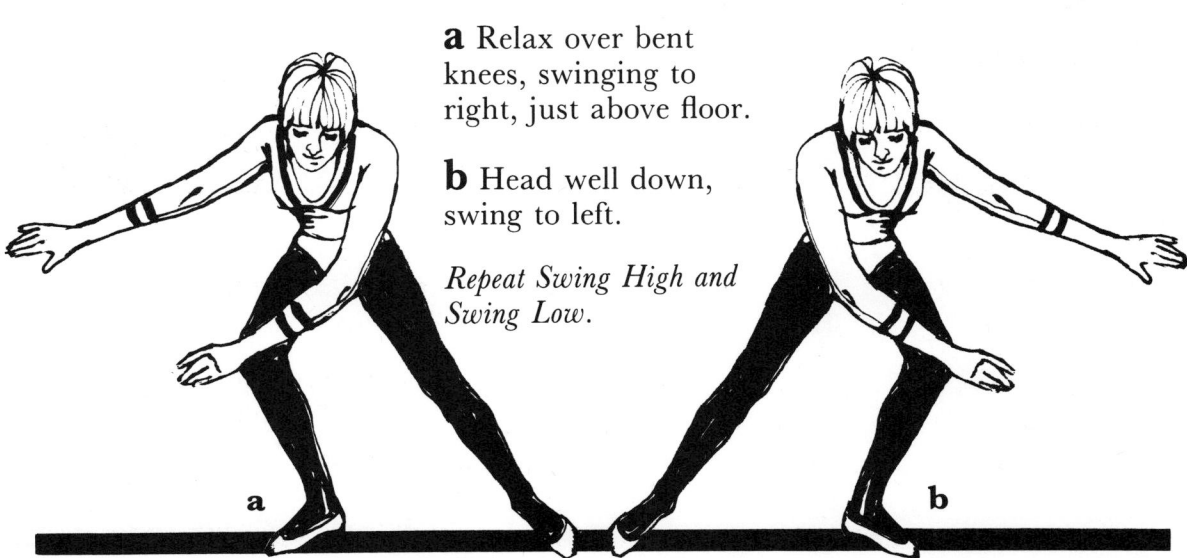

113

5 CLAP HIGH, CLAP LOW

To tone up supporting muscles and to mobilise hips.

a With left foot on seat of secure chair, stretch arms up sideways, clap twice overhead.

b Arms down sideways, head down, clap twice under knee.

Repeat high and low.

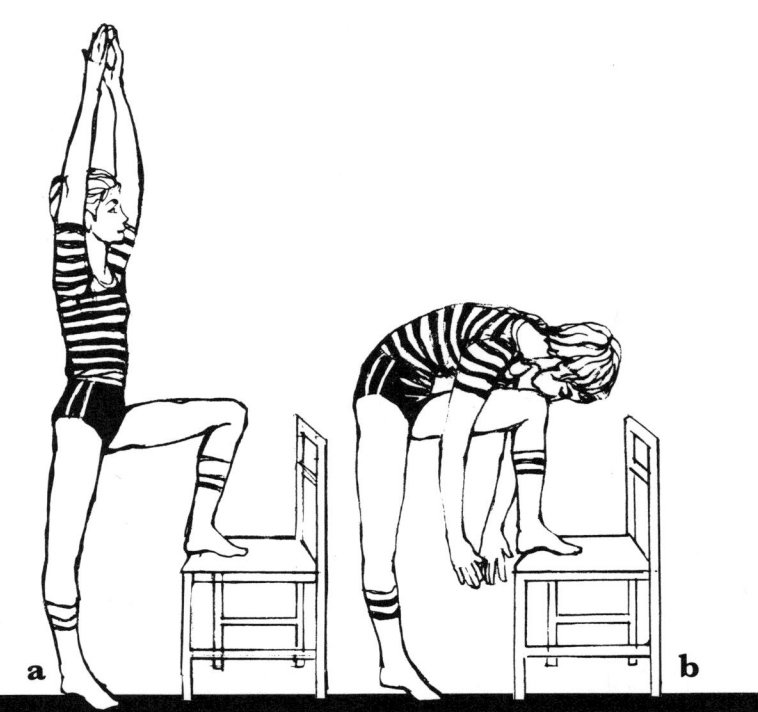

6 PULL AND FLING

A strong exercise for abdomen, arms and legs.

a With feet wide apart, sit on floor, clasp both knees and pull up close.

b Stretch feet apart and fling arms up high in a V position.

Repeat several times, and relax.

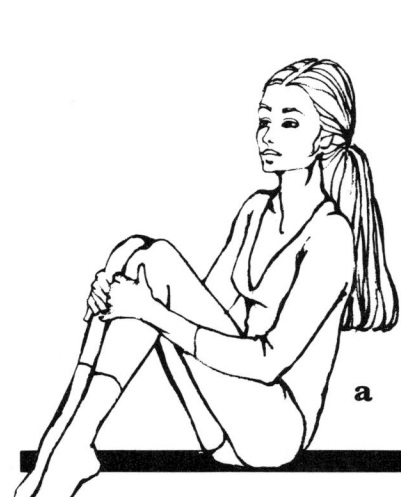

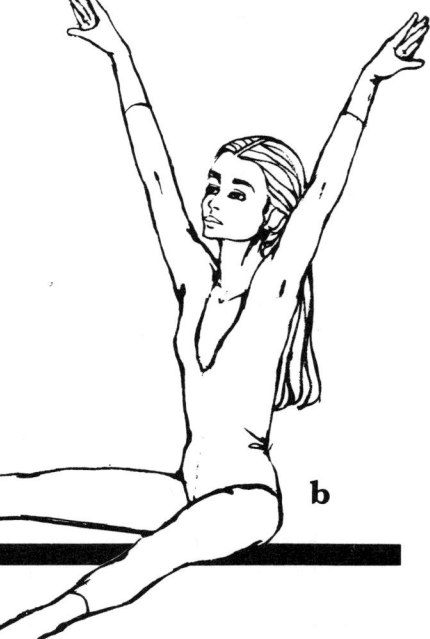

7 DIVE AND SHAKE

A top to toe slimming exercise for balance and poise.

a Feet together, raise both arms up sideways, palms facing front, thumbs touching.

b Dive down to floor, bending knees. Straighten up and raise arms overhead again. Take arms down sideways.

Repeat 4 times.

c Stand on alternate legs, shaking the other to relax it. Watch your balance.

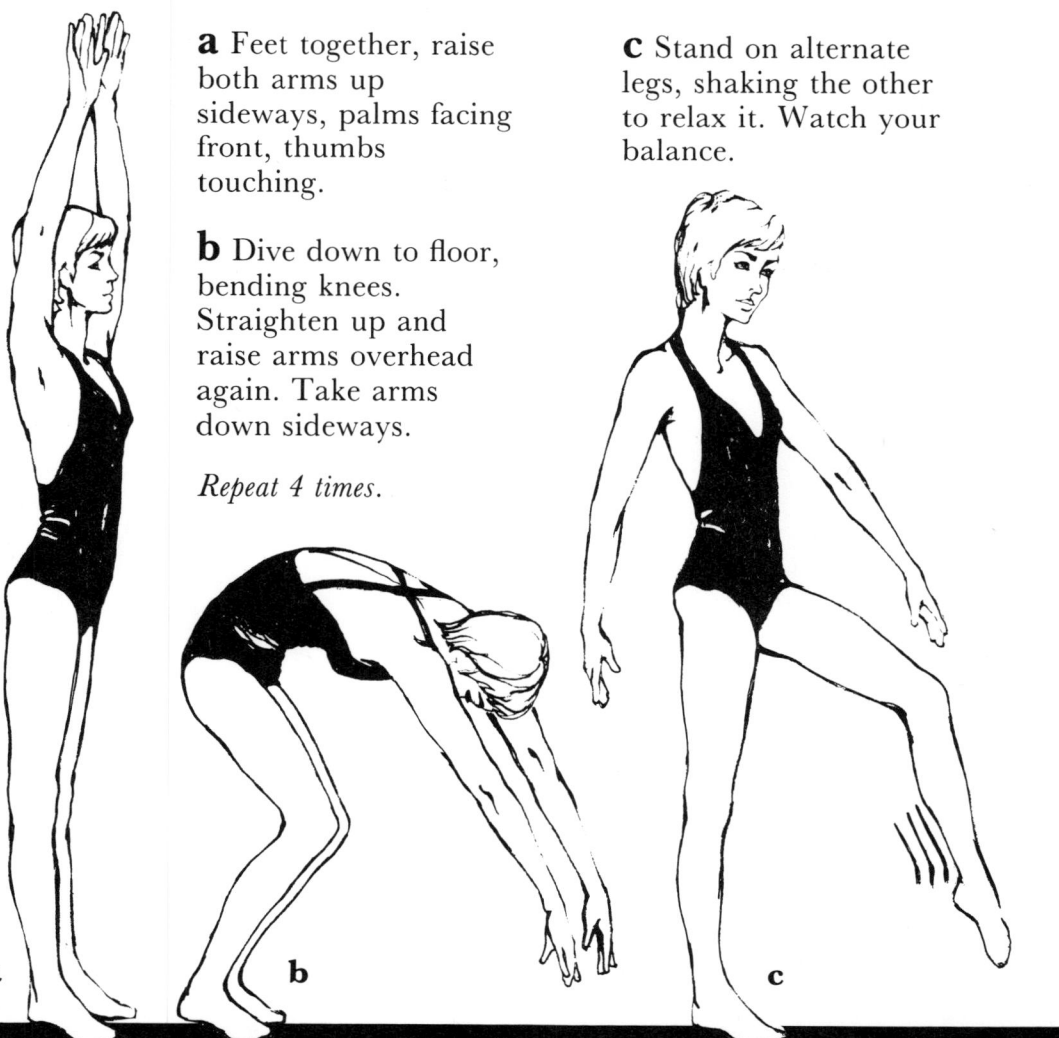

a   b   c

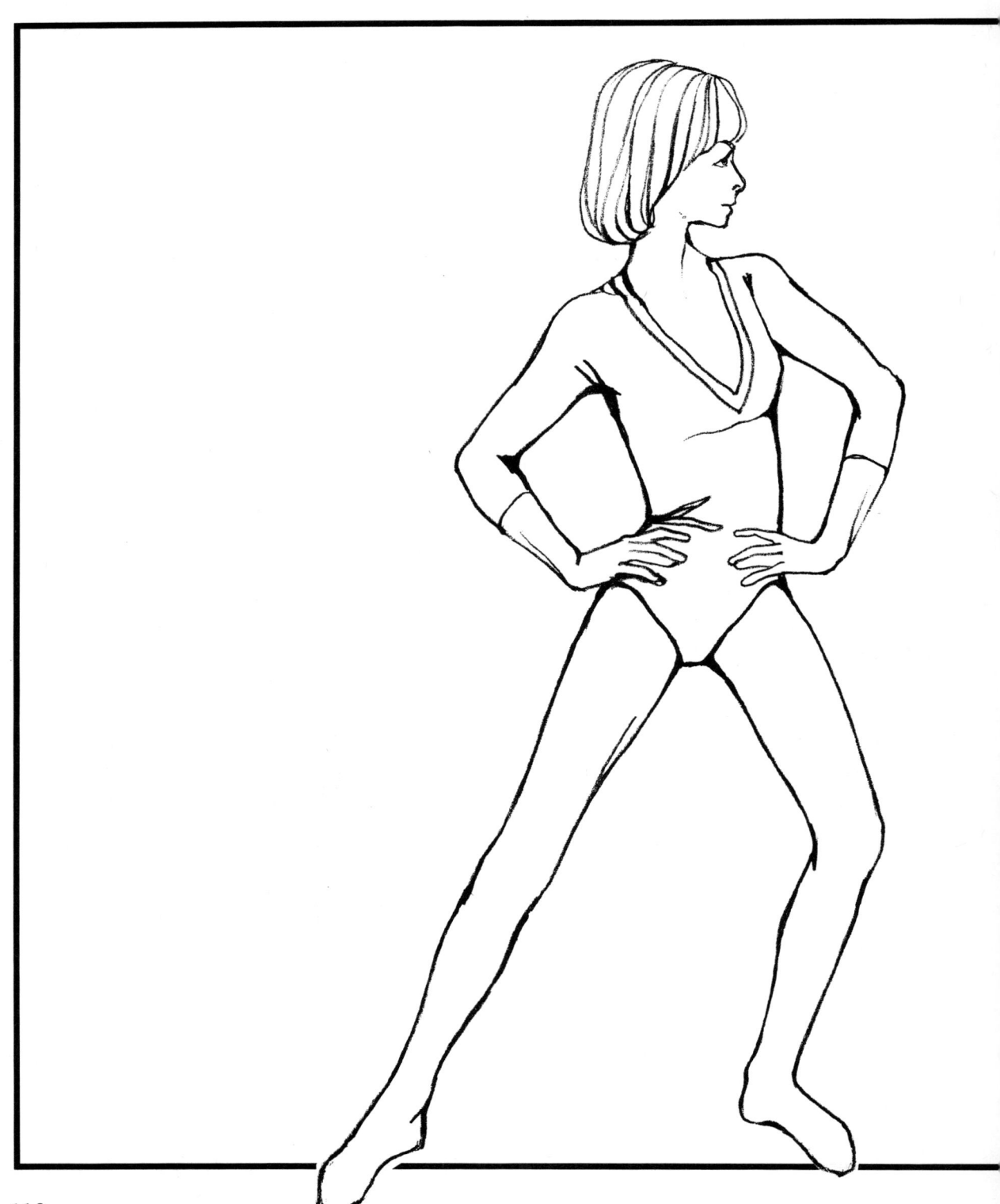

Chapter 12

Dance and keep fit

A routine for energy and elegance

If you wish to fine down your figure, increase your vitality and you love to dance, then these are your exercises. Moving this way will relieve any lassitude or tension and promote an uplift in the figure and in the frame of mind. The exercises have been designed to go with all types of dance music – from beguine to jazz – and they tend to create a party atmosphere.

The routine will encourage a relaxed, poised and elegant way of moving – the turn of the head, the graceful arm, the lift of the hip, and the pointed toe, all are there. Practise with these points in mind, and add polish to the more mundane use of muscles.

Not only will the exercises improve the appearance enormously, but they are also nice to watch, and form a ready-made keep fit demonstration. The exercises remain simple, and will give the body control and tone. It is your personality and your presentation which will make them a little different.

For music details, see Chapter 20.

1 TAP AND TIP

For co-ordination and a slim waistline.

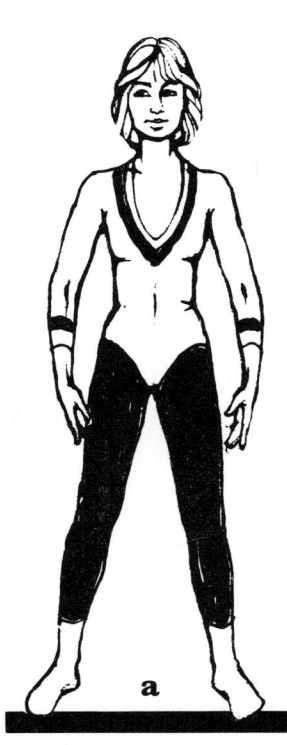

a Stand tall with feet well apart. Tap sides lightly.

b Raise both arms sideways, leaning to left, and tap fingers overhead. Tap sides again and repeat to right.

2 TOUCH TOES AND CROSS ANKLES

For graceful arm movement and strong stomach muscles.

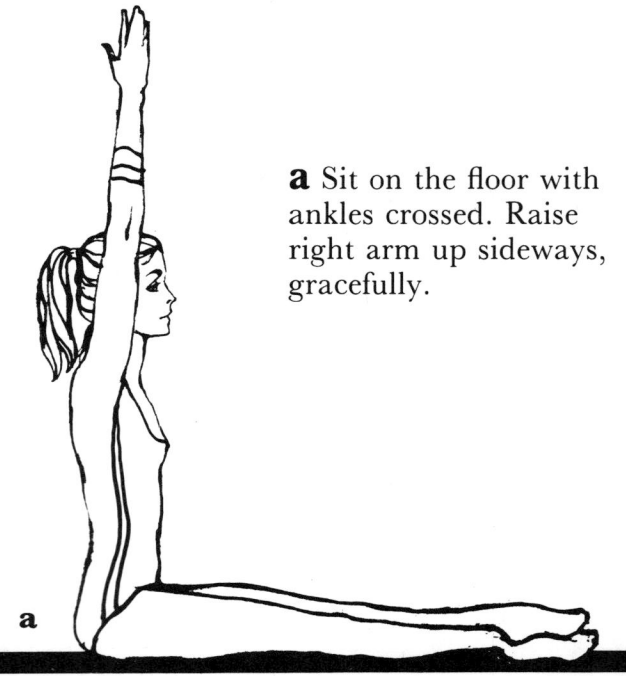

a Sit on the floor with ankles crossed. Raise right arm up sideways, gracefully.

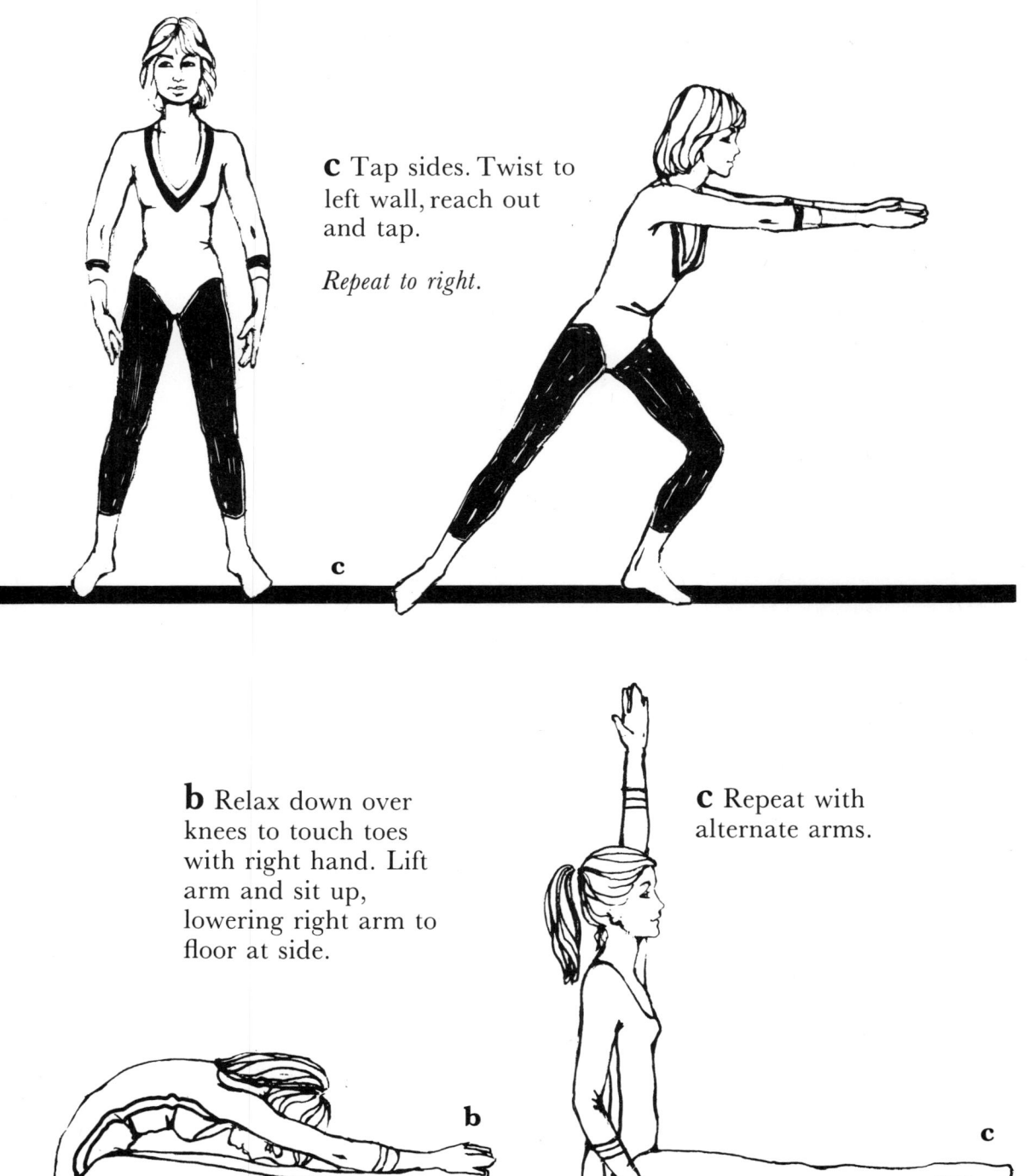

c Tap sides. Twist to left wall, reach out and tap.

Repeat to right.

b Relax down over knees to touch toes with right hand. Lift arm and sit up, lowering right arm to floor at side.

c Repeat with alternate arms.

3 SWING AND KICK (1)

A sustained movement for waistline, neckline, feet and ankles.

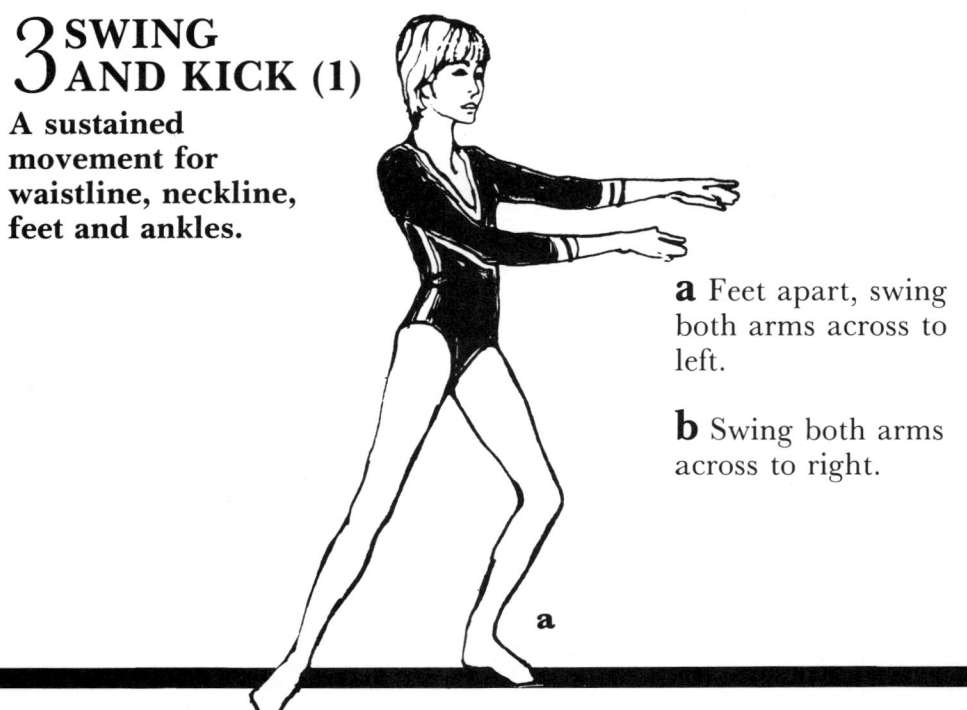

a Feet apart, swing both arms across to left.

b Swing both arms across to right.

4 SWING AND KICK (2)

To mobilise hips and train good balance.

a Step to right, kick left foot across.

b Step to left, kick right foot across.

Repeat 8 times.

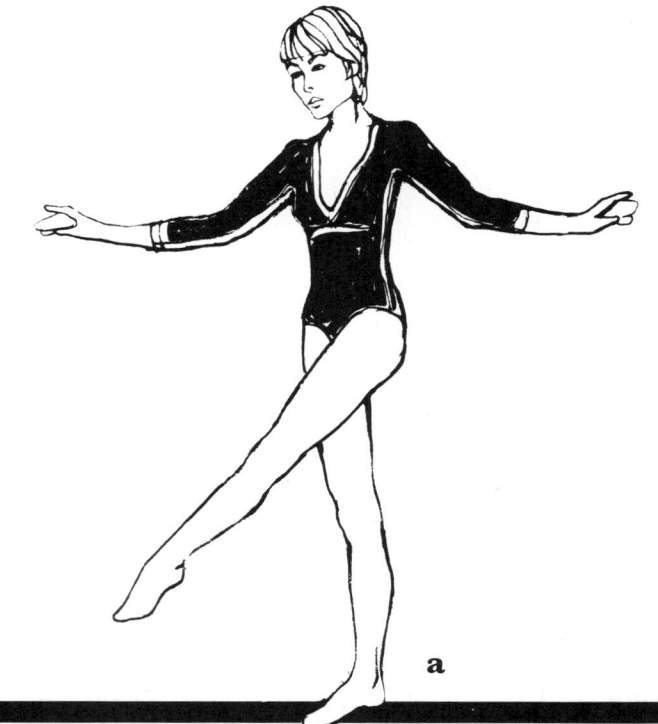

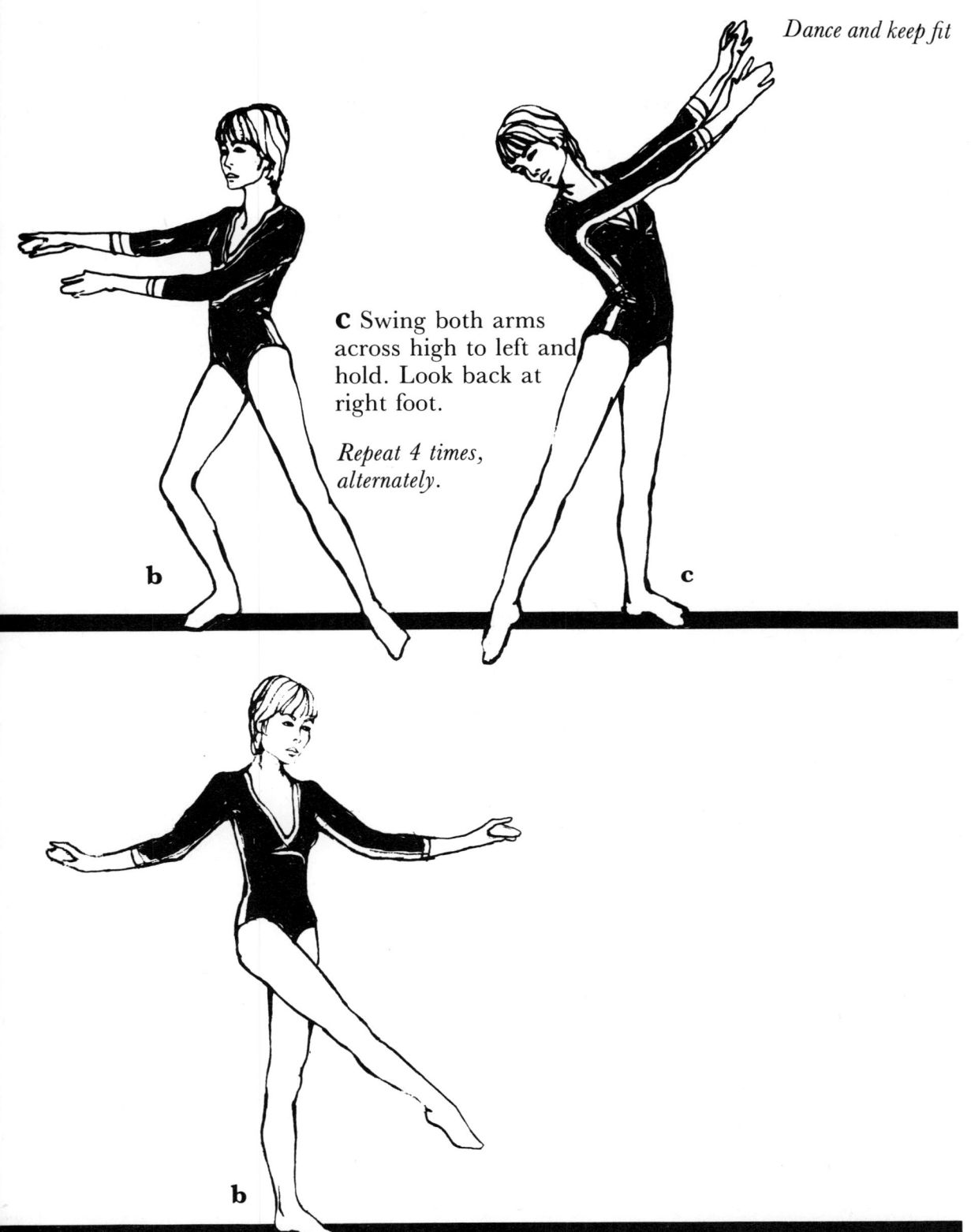

c Swing both arms across high to left and hold. Look back at right foot.

Repeat 4 times, alternately.

b

c

b

5 BEGUINE (1)

For uplift, grace, poise and figure control.

a Feet apart, raise both arms forward and up overhead. Count eight.

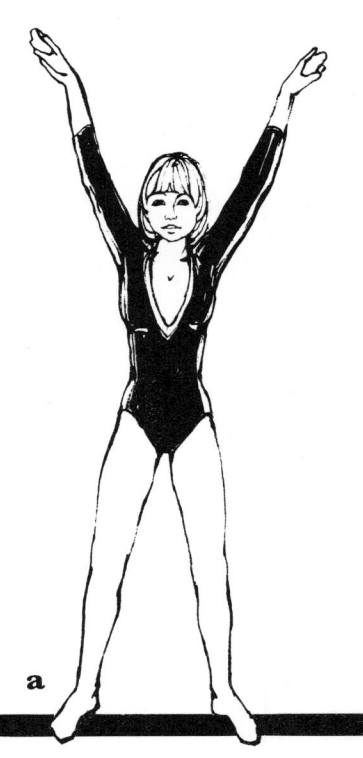

a

6 BEGUINE (2)

For hipline and good posture.

a Raise left arm up and bend sideways to right.

b Raise right arm up and bend sideways to left.

Repeat alternately 4 times.

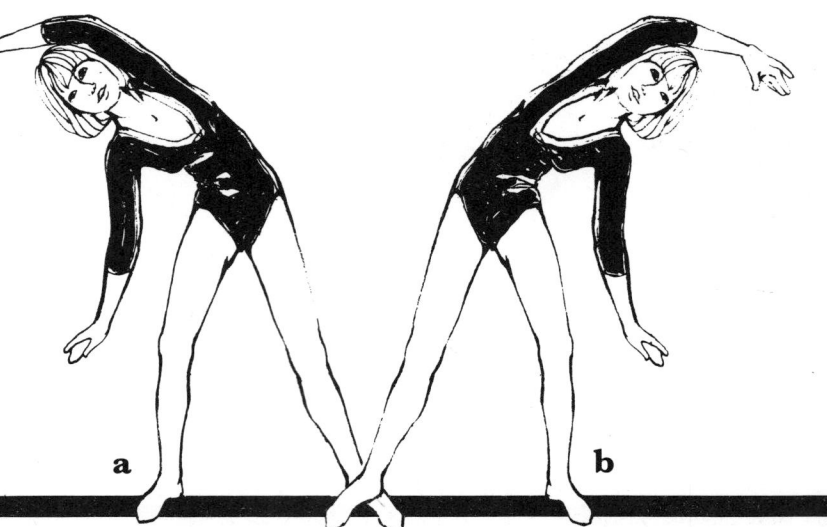

a   **b**

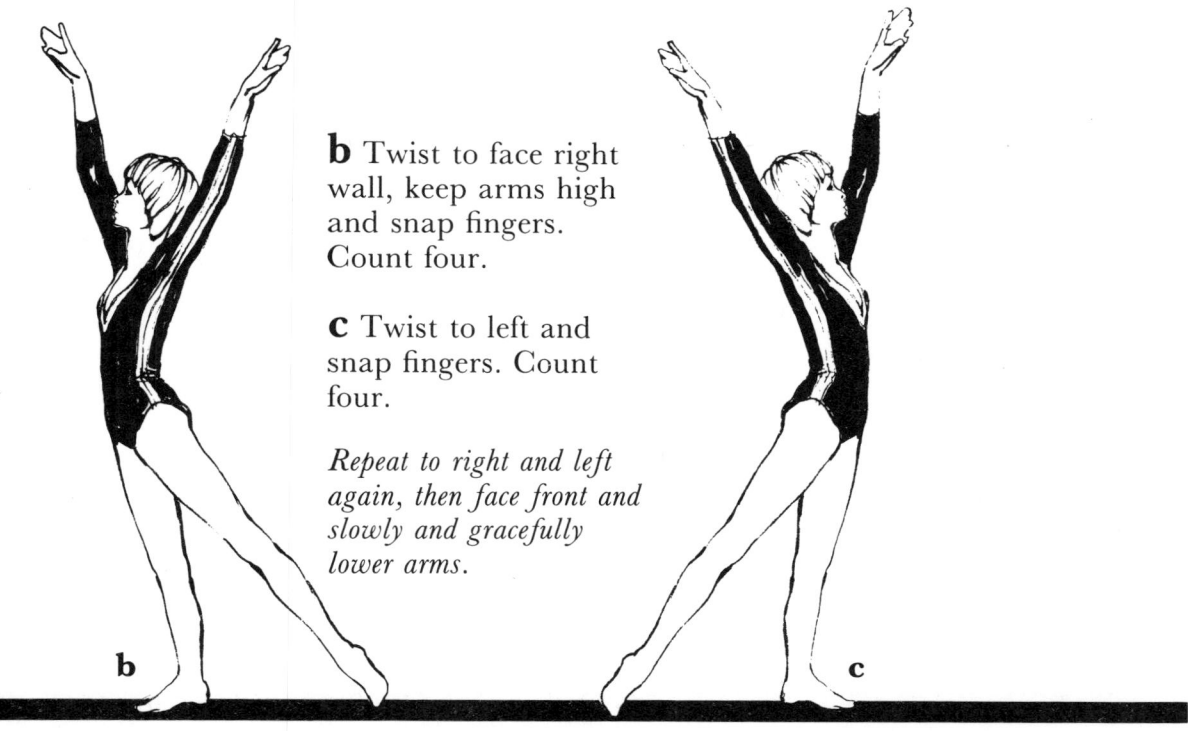

b Twist to face right wall, keep arms high and snap fingers. Count four.

c Twist to left and snap fingers. Count four.

Repeat to right and left again, then face front and slowly and gracefully lower arms.

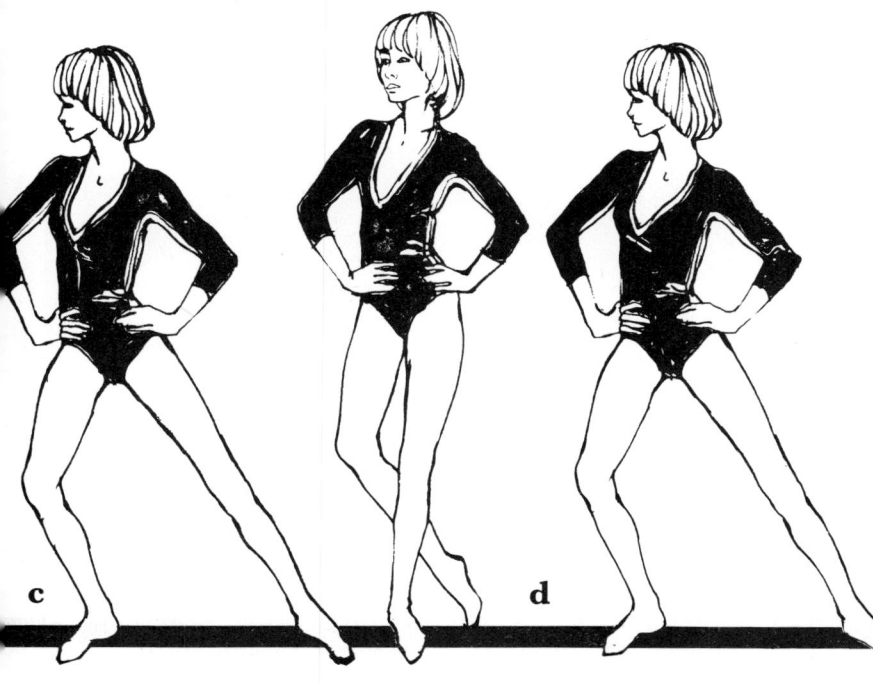

c With hands on hips step sideways with right foot, turn head to right.

d Step across with left foot. Step sideways again with right foot and bring left to right and close as in tango step.

Repeat 4 times, alternately to right and left.

123

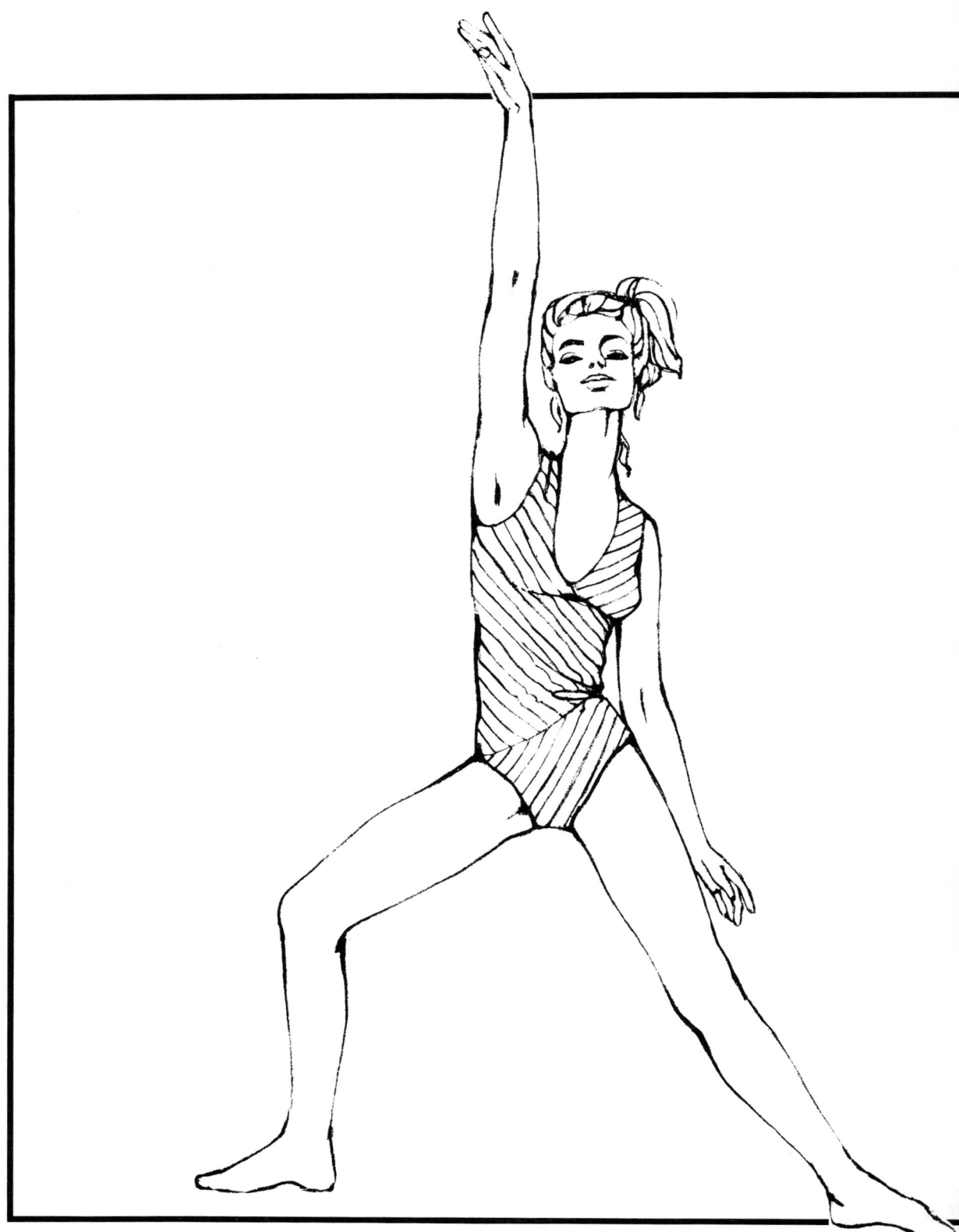

124

Chapter 13

Dance mobility

Dance disco – the keep fit way

I have included three dance mobility routines – Dance Disco, Rocket Routine and Dance Quartet – because this kind of movement, based on dance, is popular with everyone and is definitely not restricted to the young.

Disco music is modern; it has a steady beat but is not as fast as some pop music. The music is not 'background' as the steps in Dance Disco change with the musical phrases. The routine is recorded on the BBC record 'Dance and Keep Fit' (see Chapter 20).

The Rocket Routine can be practised to pop music. These exercises are meant to be taken at a faster pace than usual, as the movements are small and less sustained. They are my tonic exercises – exhilarating, fun to do and excellent for circulation, mobility and co-ordination. Because of the pace and the importance of the beat, thinking quickly is a must, and the repetitions will mean that you have to work hard. But do not overdo it. If you get out of breath, stop. This is not a specific treatment for the heart and lungs; it is just keeping fit to rhythm, based on dance. Always start gently and warm up gradually to slower music. The important point when choosing music is to select a simple and straightforward arrangement. If it is catchy and easy to remember, it will be easy to dance to.

The Dance Quartet movements test balance and help to slim the waistline. The routine need not be practised to very fast music, but it must be continuous and have a bright tempo.

DANCE DISCO

The steps are simple but rely on a change of weight for a smooth way of moving. Step 1 encourages a light and balanced way of walking; Step 2 is good for continuity and co-ordination; Step 3 trains concentration and memory; and Step 4 gives a strong final bend and stretch. If balance is a problem, this last step can be done with a partner, or holding on to a firm support.

Step 1

a Take 4 steps forward, starting with right foot.

b Step to right and close feet, weight remaining on right foot.

c Step to left and close feet, weight remaining on left foot.

Step 2

d Step sideways to right with right foot.

e Step across with left foot.

f Step right again.

g Turn towards left wall and kick with left leg.

Repeat whole step 8 times, starting with alternate feet.

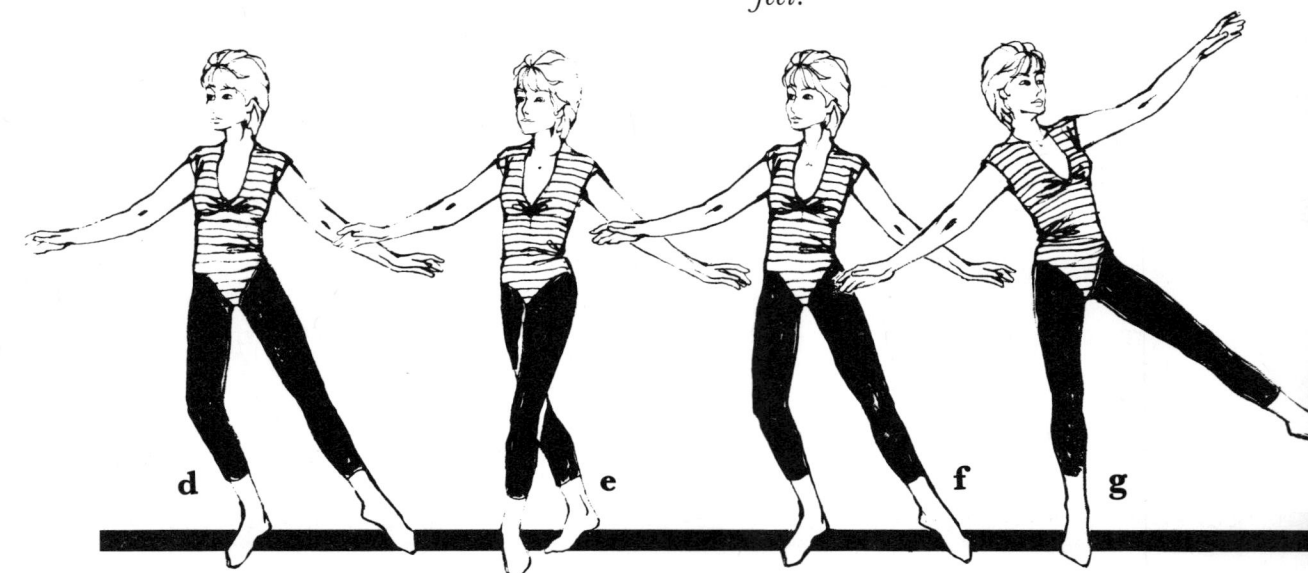

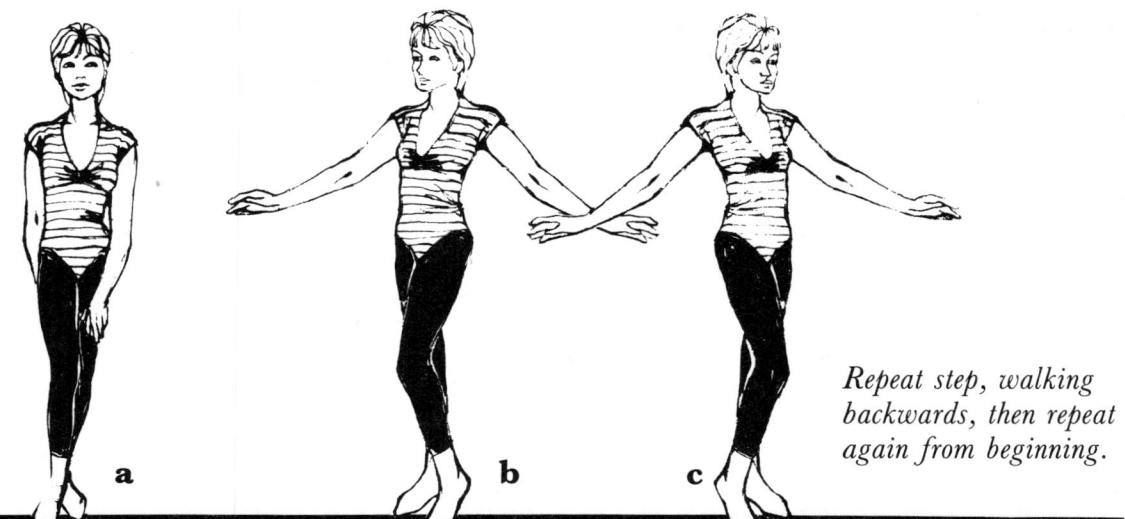

a   b   c

Repeat step, walking backwards, then repeat again from beginning.

Step 3

h Step right and close.

i Step left and close, and step twice to right.

Repeat alternately 4 times.

Step 4

j Step to right, raise left knee and cross to right.

k Quickly stretch left leg down to side on toe.

Repeat with alternate legs, 8 times in all.

Final Step

Towards end of routine, the bend and stretch (j and k) can be done twice each way instead of once.

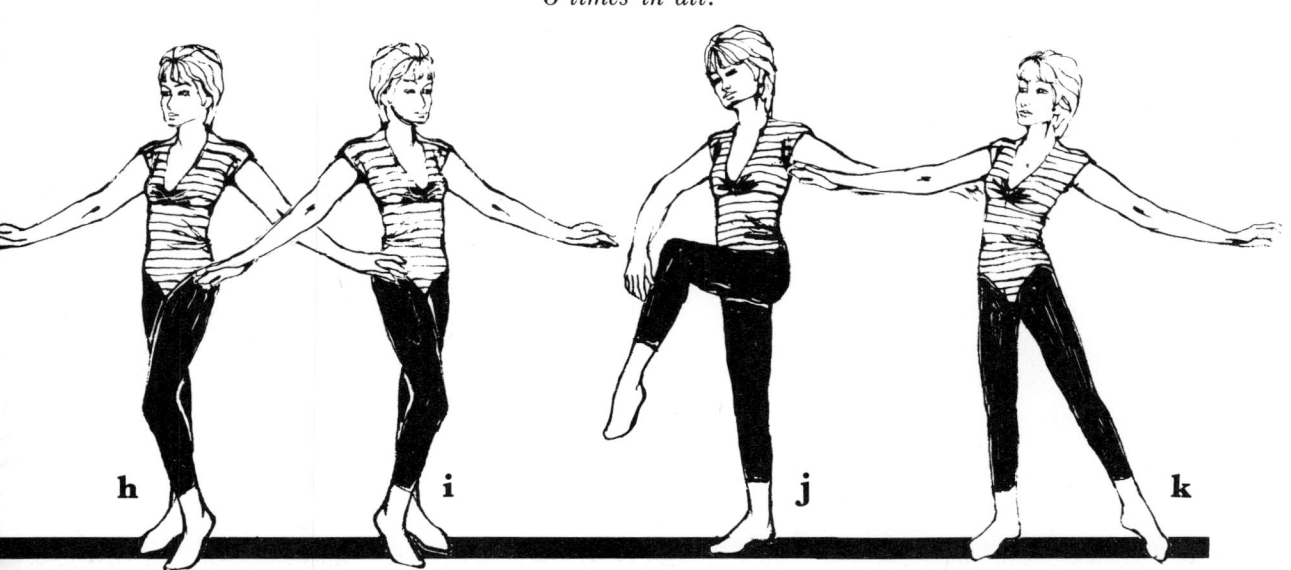

h   i   j   k

ROCKET ROUTINE

Be sure to start the routine with your feet wide apart, and repeat Steps 1 to 4 four times. Bend your knees deeply each time you touch the floor, and drop very gently on to your knees in Step 5. From then on, take your time – a simple break (Step 7), and then the big stretch to finish.

PART 1
Step 1

Feet well apart. On count of one, bend elbows and press palms together.

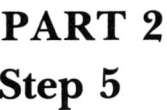

PART 2
Step 5

Move hands forward and kneel.

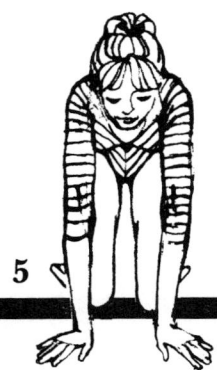

Step 6

Kneel up. Make a fist with both hands and tap them together twice in front and twice behind.

Repeat as required.

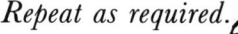

Step 2

On count of two,
stretch both arms
straight up over head.

Step 3

On count of three,
bring arms down
sideways, in
continuous movement.

Step 4

On count of four, drop
quickly down towards
feet, hands to floor.

*Repeat the whole of Part
1 four times, and on last
drop, stay down.*

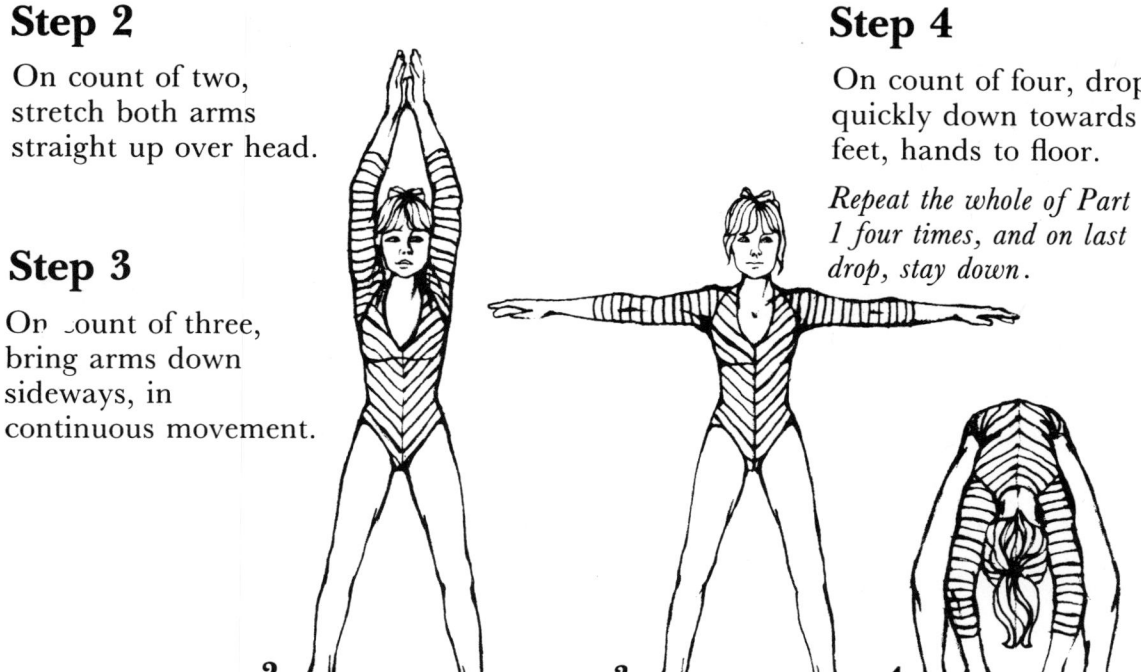

Step 7

Arms out to side,
ready for heel touch.

Step 8

Lean back gently to
touch heels with
alternate hands.

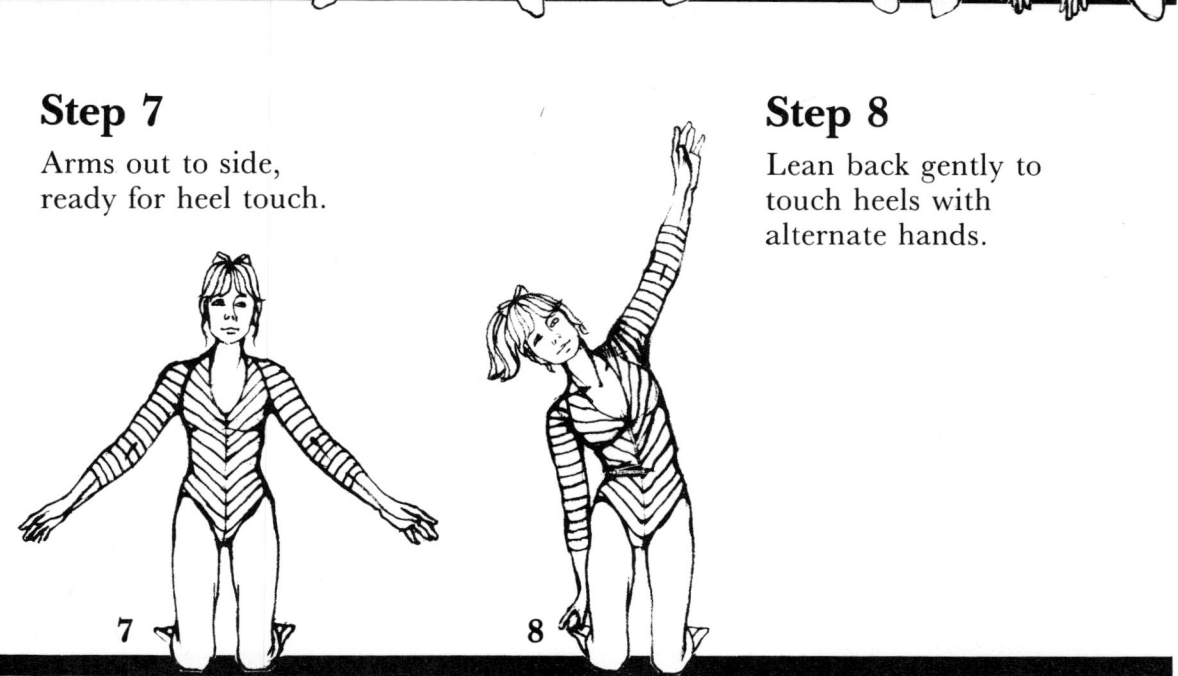

DANCE QUARTET

Lift the knee as high as possible in Step 1 to mobilise the hip joint, giving a bigger range of movement. It is important to step to the side with one foot before raising the other knee, as this gives a tidy start on the first beat of the bar and allows time for a high lift of the knee. Steps 1, 2 and 3 are repeated eight times. Hold the final lunge to make a strong finish.

Stand tall with feet together.

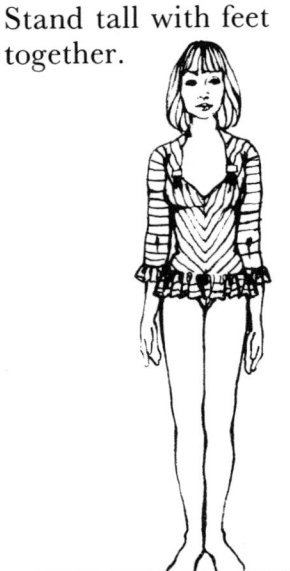

Step 2

Step sideways to right, raising left knee high. Clap under knee.

Repeat alternately 8 times.

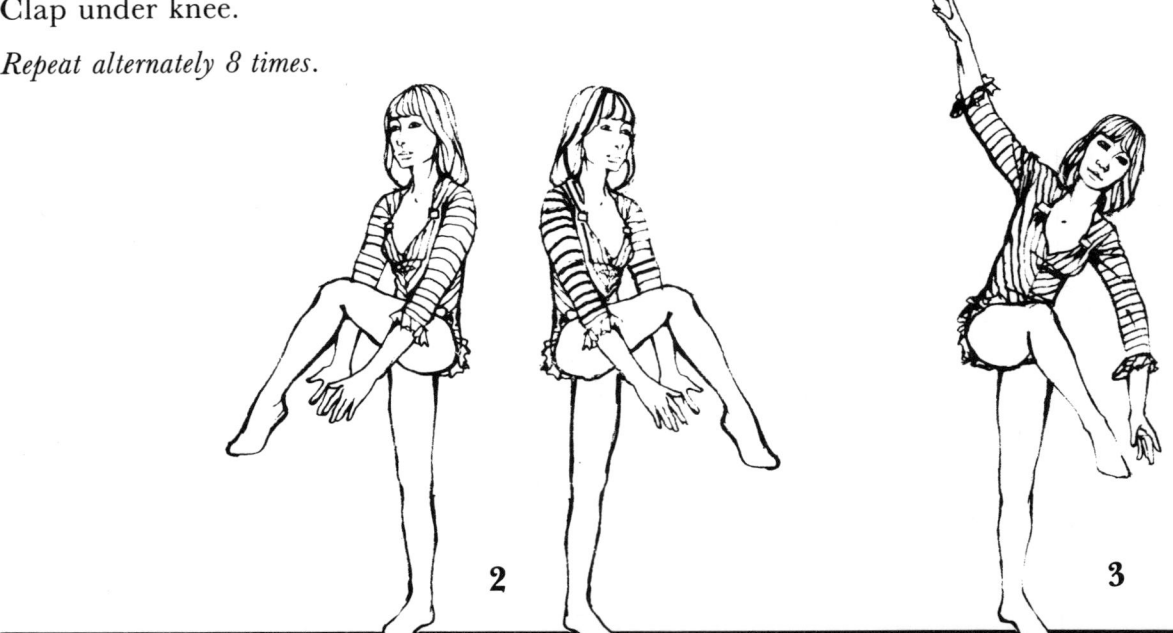

2

3

Step 1

Step sideways to right, raising left knee up and across to touch right elbow.

Repeat alternately 8 times.

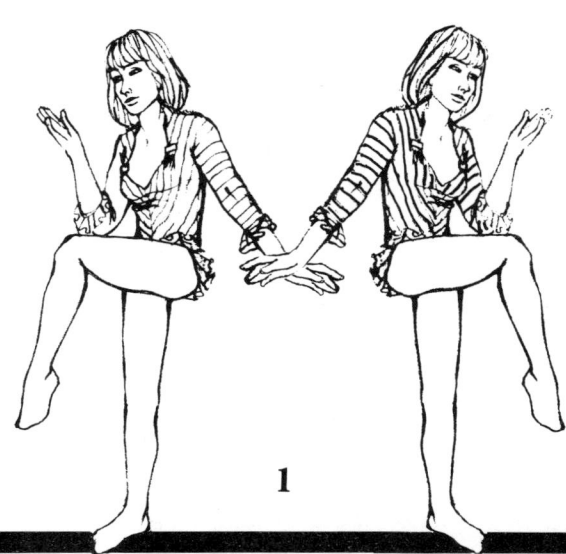

Step 3

Step sideways to right, raising left foot across in front. Touch toes with right hand, stretching left arm to aid balance.

Repeat alternately 8 times.

Step 4

Take big step sideways to right, stretching right arm up close beside head. Return and close feet.

Repeat to left, and as often as required.

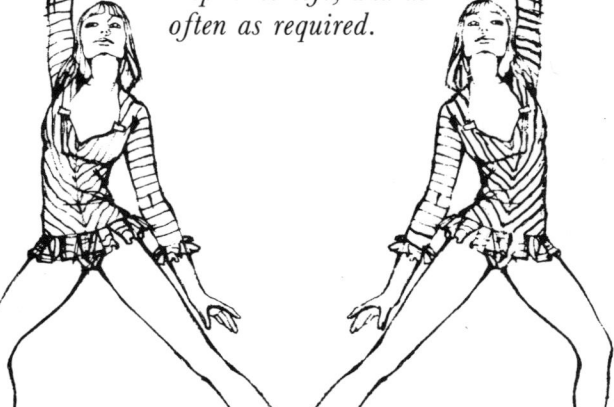

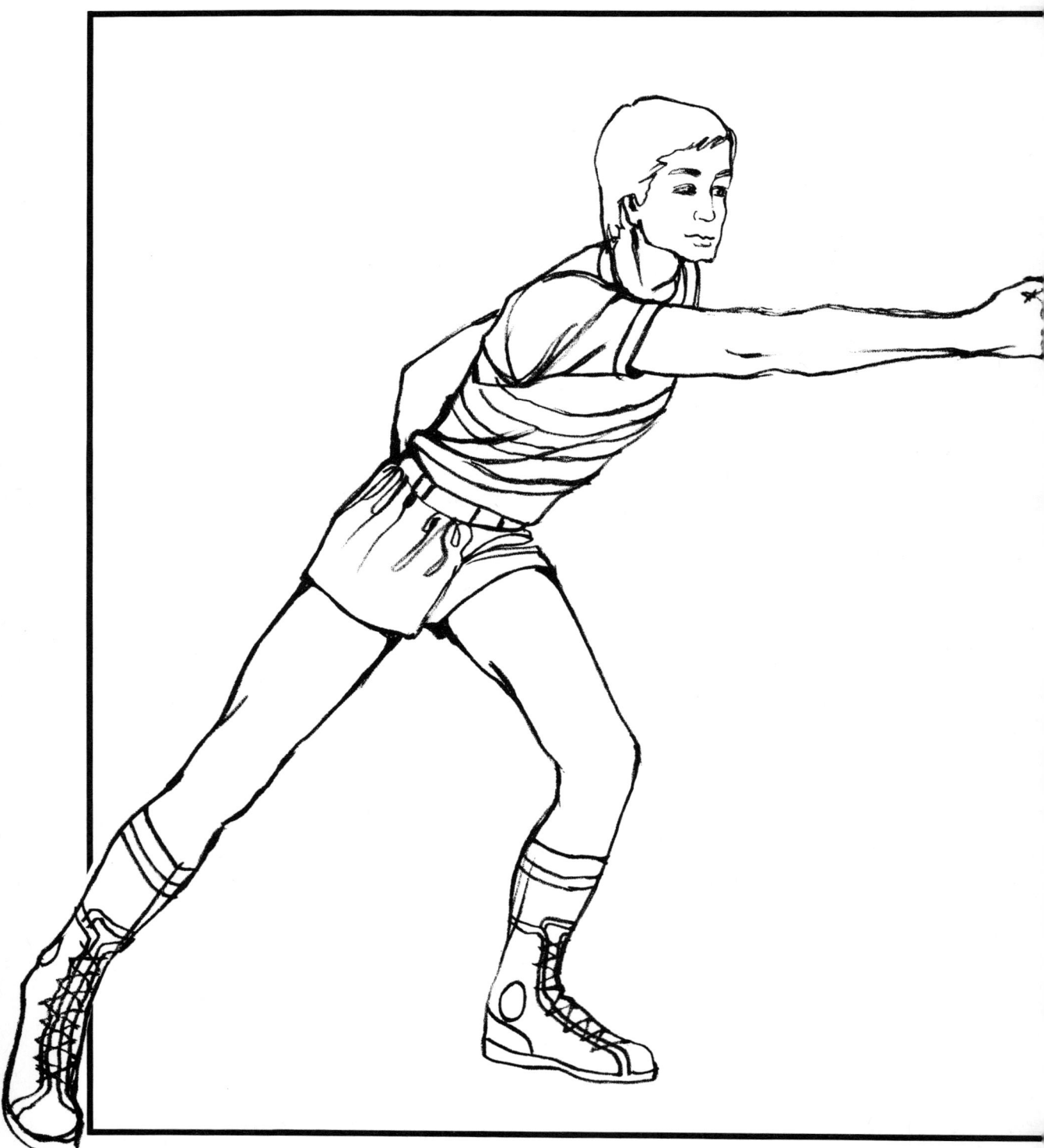

Chapter 14

Mainly for men

A routine to increase energy, strength and mobility

An increasing number of men are realising that if they wish to stay young and active all their lives, they cannot allow their muscles to become slack or their joints to set. If you are interested in keeping fit, I strongly recommend the following conditioning exercises. They are not time-consuming and can slot quite easily into daily life. The movements are basic and probably familiar, but they will increase energy, strength and mobility if practised regularly. Do the exercises in the order given, as the first three serve as a warm-up.

If you sit at a desk or have a sedentary job, be sure not to miss exercise 7, Swing and Stretch. It is a comprehensive antidote to a fixed position. If you are concerned about stomach muscles, the two floor exercises will attend to these. The chair exercises are good for waists, thighs and stomach muscles.

Always be conscious that the habit of standing tall will help you to retain your present height, and that practising the backstroke exercise from Chapter 16, Morning Choice, will prevent round shoulders. Many of the exercises in other chapters are suitable for both men and women.

1 THE PUSHAWAY

For shoulders and back muscles, to increase strength and flexibility.

a Lean against a wall at arm's length. Slowly press forward, chest to wall, bending elbows.

b Push away, return to start.

Repeat.

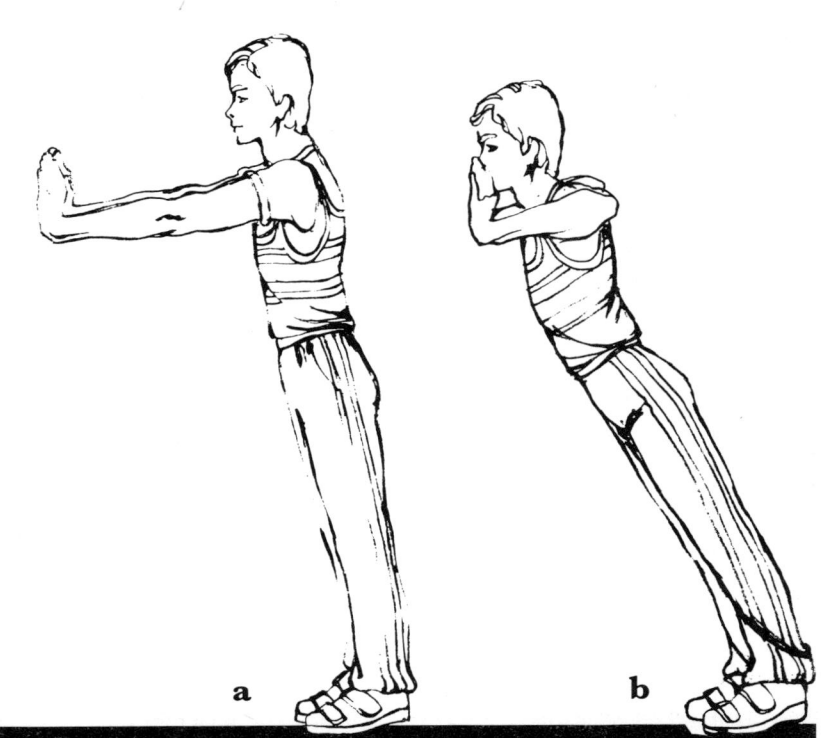

a   b

2 ROLL AROUND

To counteract stiffness and tension in the neck.

Move head gently in all directions, looking around the room.

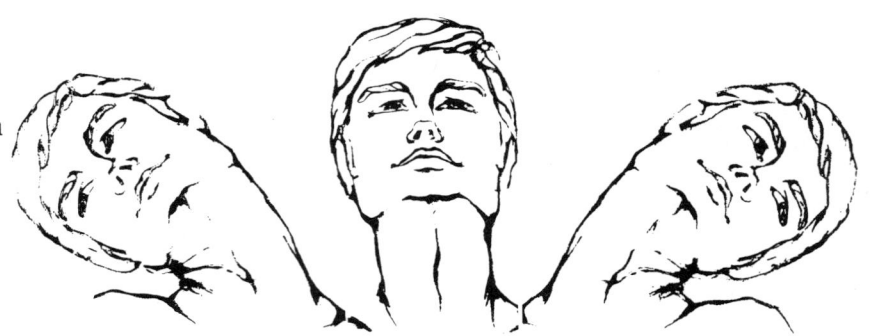

3 EASY DOES IT

To loosen up stiff knees, to strengthen leg muscles and to save the back.

a With both hands, support yourself securely. Bend knees deeply.

b Straighten up slowly with straight back.

Repeat.

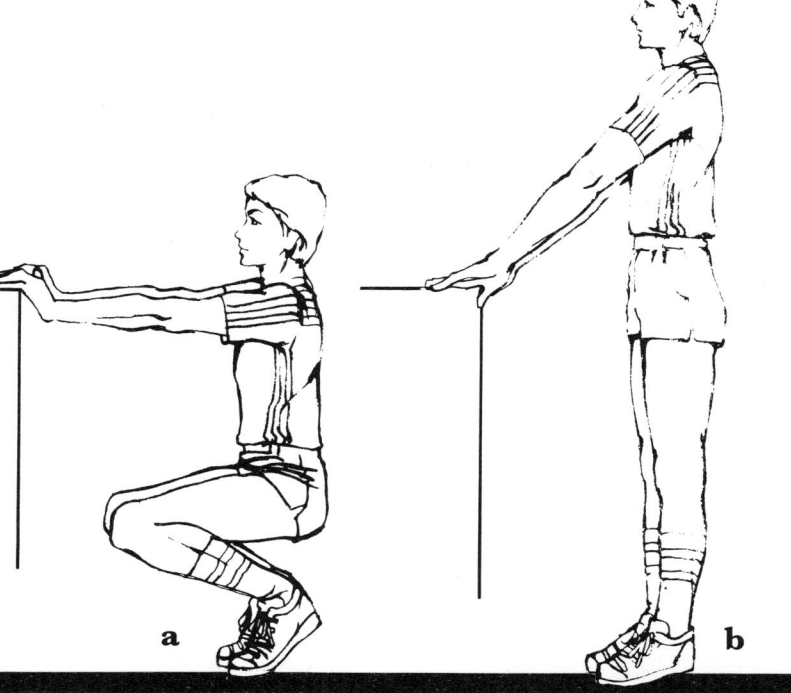

4 LEG LIFT BEHIND

To strengthen back muscles.

a Lying on stomach, raise left leg slowly, and lower.

b Raise right leg slowly, and lower.

Repeat.

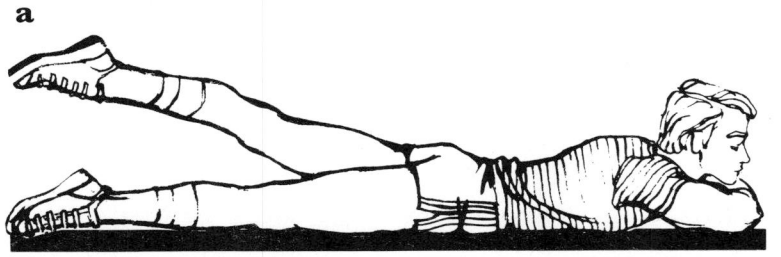

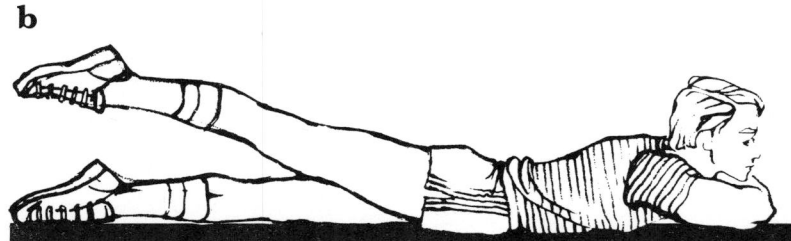

135

5 LEG LIFT

To tone slack stomach muscles.

a Lying on back, raise left leg, and lower.

Repeat with right leg. Practise alternately.

b When ready, raise both legs at same time. Hold, and lower.

Repeat.

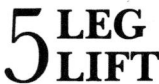

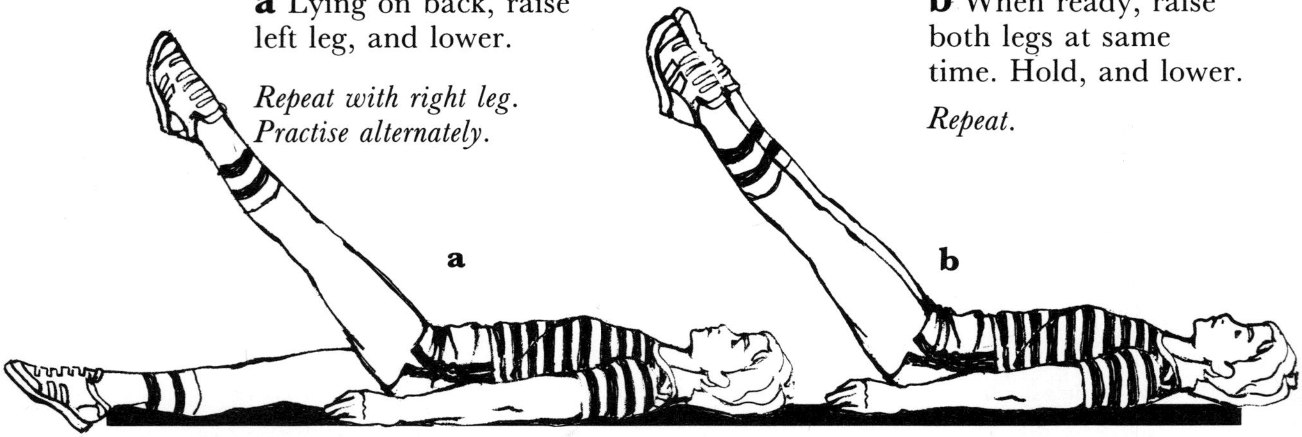

6 PUNCH

To mobilise shoulders, upper back and waist areas.

a With weight on right foot, bend right arm and make fist. Pull back for start.

b Straighten arm and punch across towards left wall. Then twist to right and punch to right wall.

Repeat, keeping movement continuous.

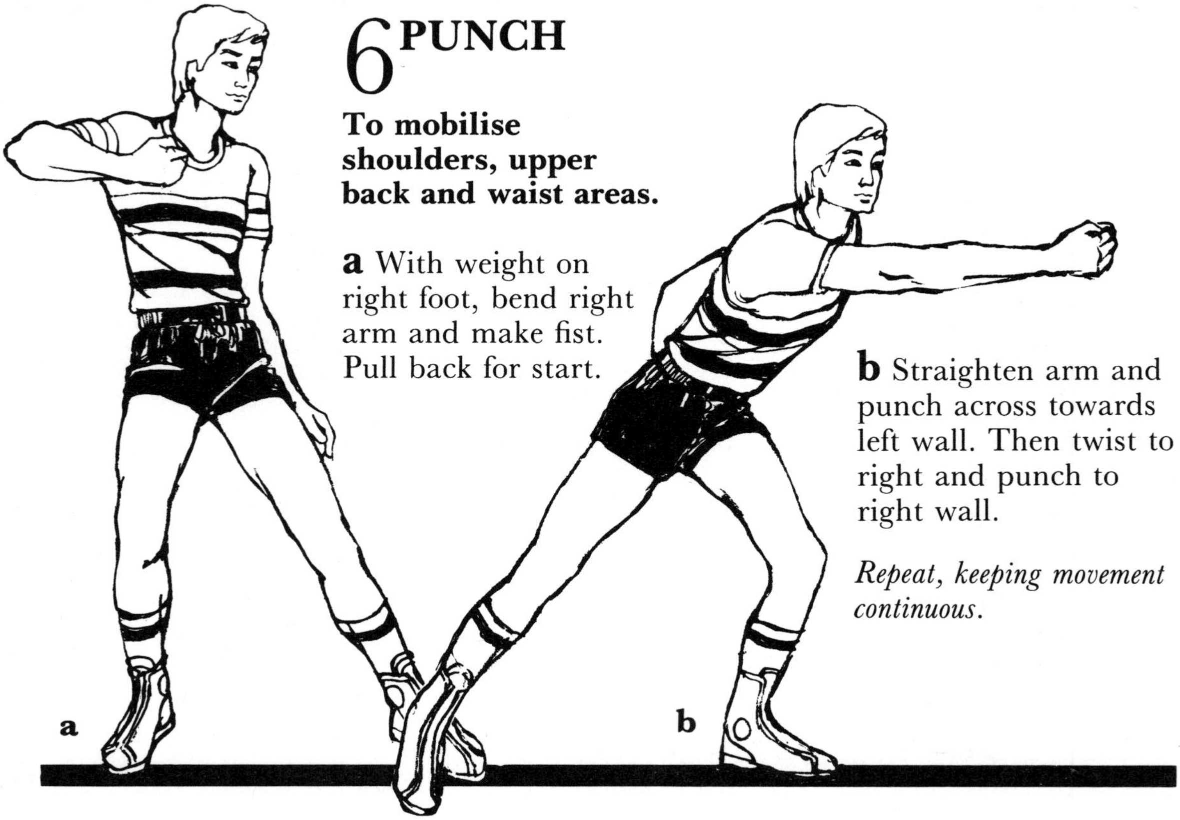

7 SWING AND STRETCH

A comprehensive exercise for stomach muscles, knees and good posture.

a With feet together, stretch both arms forwards and up above head.

b Swing forward, down, and back, head well down over knees.

c Swing arms forward and up, bending elbows, hands to shoulders.

Repeat.

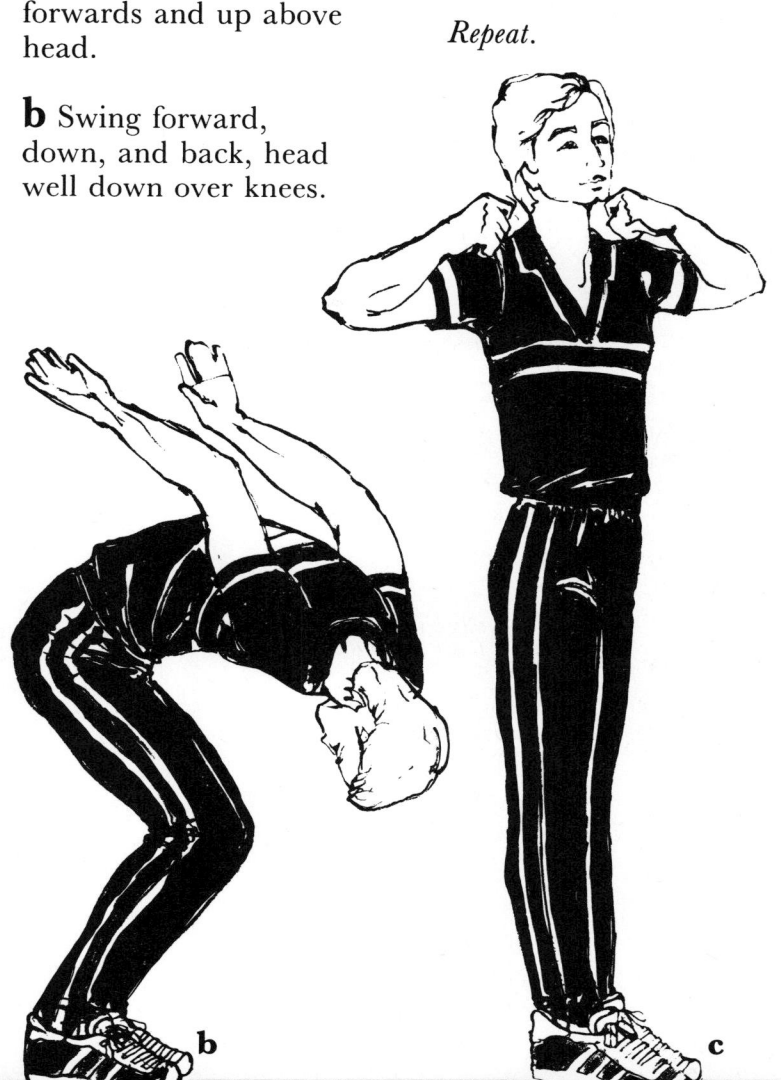

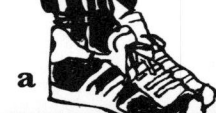

8 TRIMMING TWISTS

To prevent a thickening waistline.

a Sit astride chair, facing back. Swing both arms round to right.

b Swing both arms round to left.

Repeat.

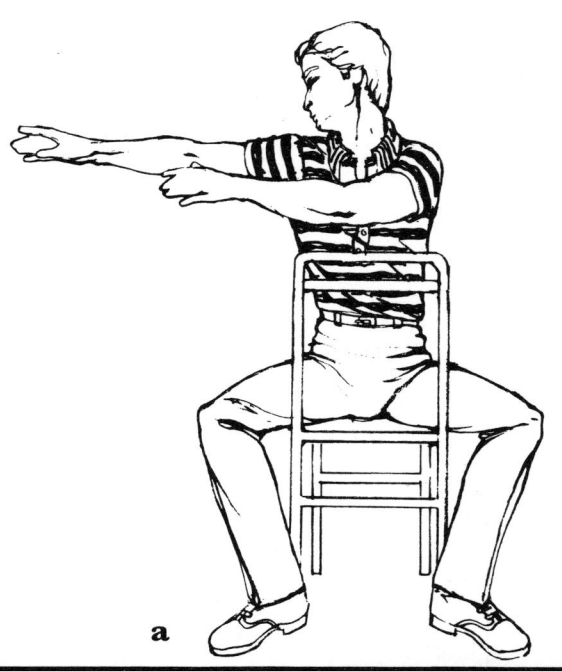

a

9 STRETCH AND FLING

To strengthen legs, thighs and stomach muscles.

a Sit astride chair, facing back. Grip chair back with hands.

b Lift legs to chair seat height. Hold, and lower to floor.

c As a progression, fling both arms high at same time as leg lift. Hold, and lower.

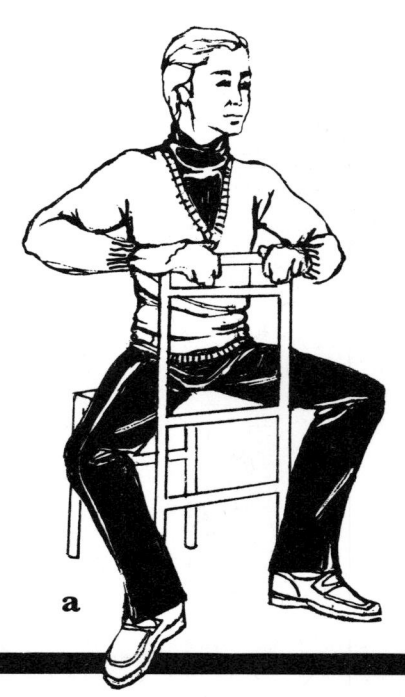

a

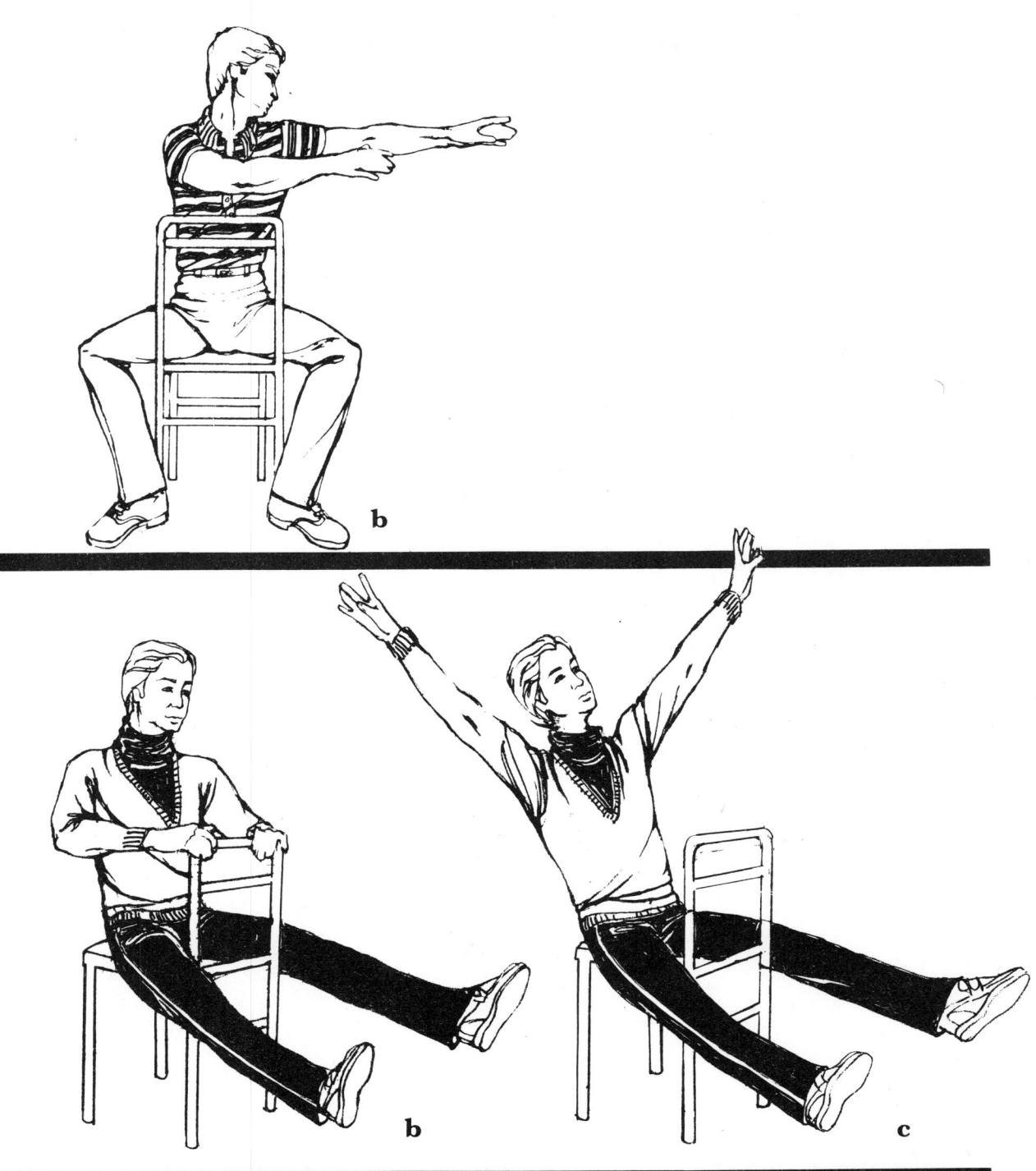

b

b

c

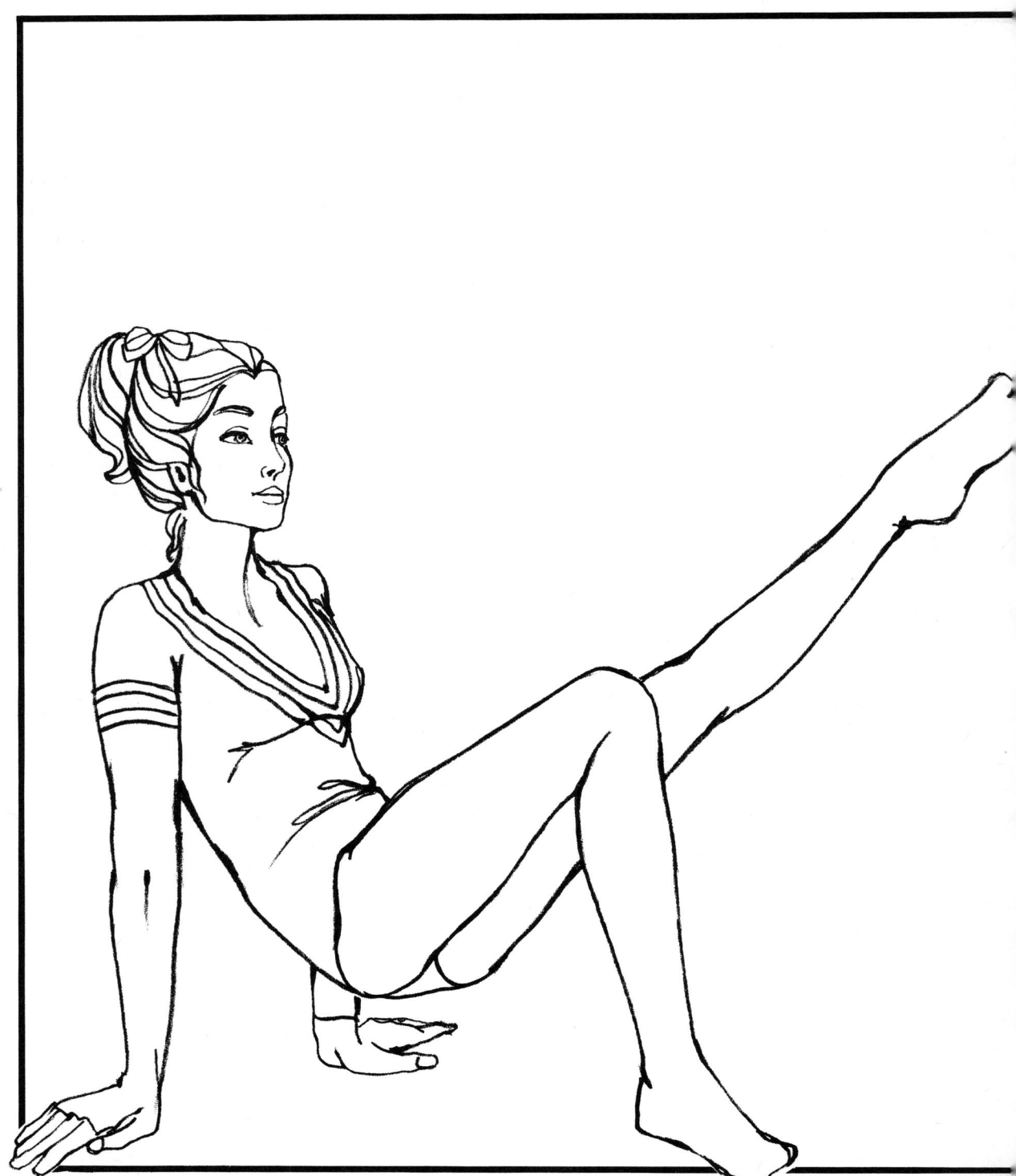

Chapter 15

Move more!

A selection of advanced exercises

These exercises form a natural progression from those in Chapters 9 to 12, and they will present no difficulty for anyone accustomed to moving in this way. I would stress, however, that to derive the maximum benefit from your practice, a certain amount of exercise experience is required. This can be gained by working through the earlier chapters and thoroughly absorbing the basic movements.

The purpose of this chapter is to broaden the whole concept of a normal keep fit exercise, and to encourage the body to move to its fullest capacity. The exercises are designed to make you think in terms of using more space, and allowing the movements to flow one into the other. It is important to get the 'feel' of moving in a more fluid way, to co-ordinate these lifts and sweeps, and to be in complete control of the body. In this way you will gain the poise, confidence and grace for which you work. Exercises 8 to 11 become more acrobatic and aim at improving strength and agility as well as the figure.

When choosing suitable music, the broad rule is move to melody and exercise to beat.

1 SWEEP AND STRETCH

For maximum movement throughout the body, including chest, back and shoulders, waistline and hips.

a Take a big step to left, raising left arm up sideways.

b Sweep left arm across overhead to right, bending right knee.

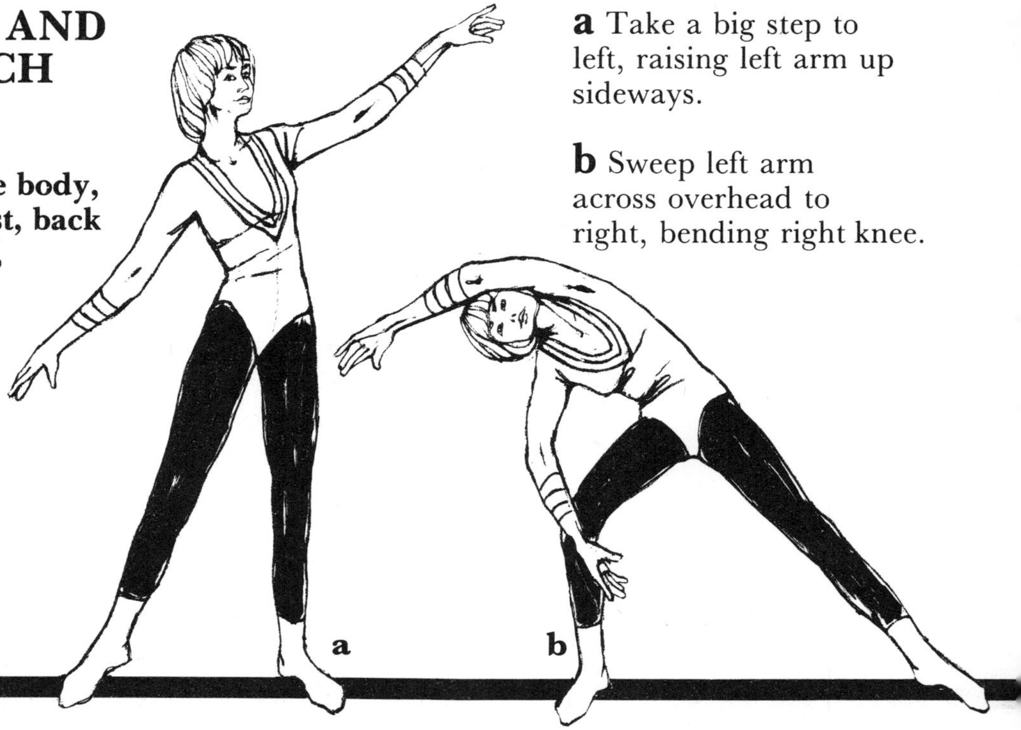

2 FULL BODY CIRCLE

A rotary exercise to give elasticity to the figure and to strengthen abdominal muscles.

a With feet apart, drop down to right foot, arms relaxed, head down.

b Sweep both arms across left foot, beginning the upward stretch.

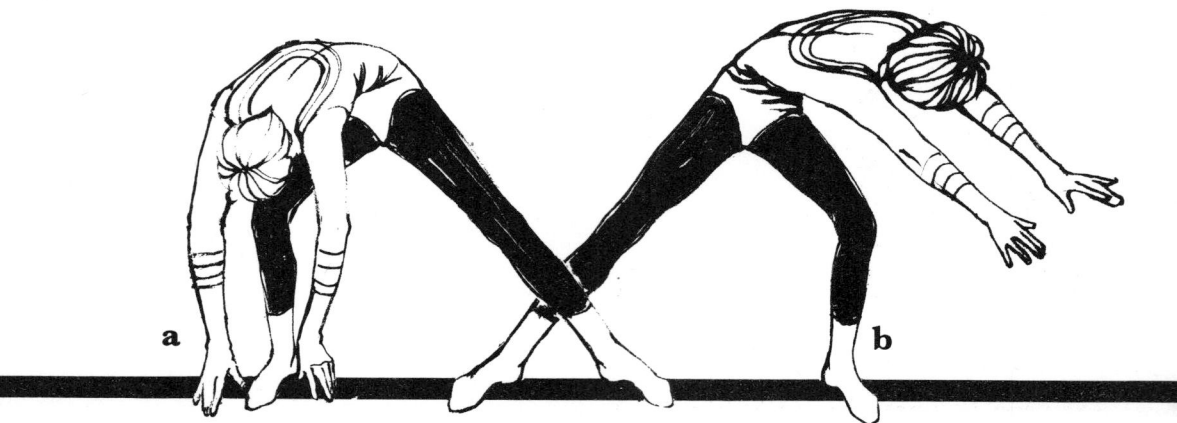

c Sweep left arm back overhead and stretch towards left wall, taking weight over to left foot.

Repeat b and c sweeps.

d Relax and drop down to touch right foot with left hand. Slowly uncurl, stand tall.

Repeat from a, stepping to the right. Then go straight to exercise 2.

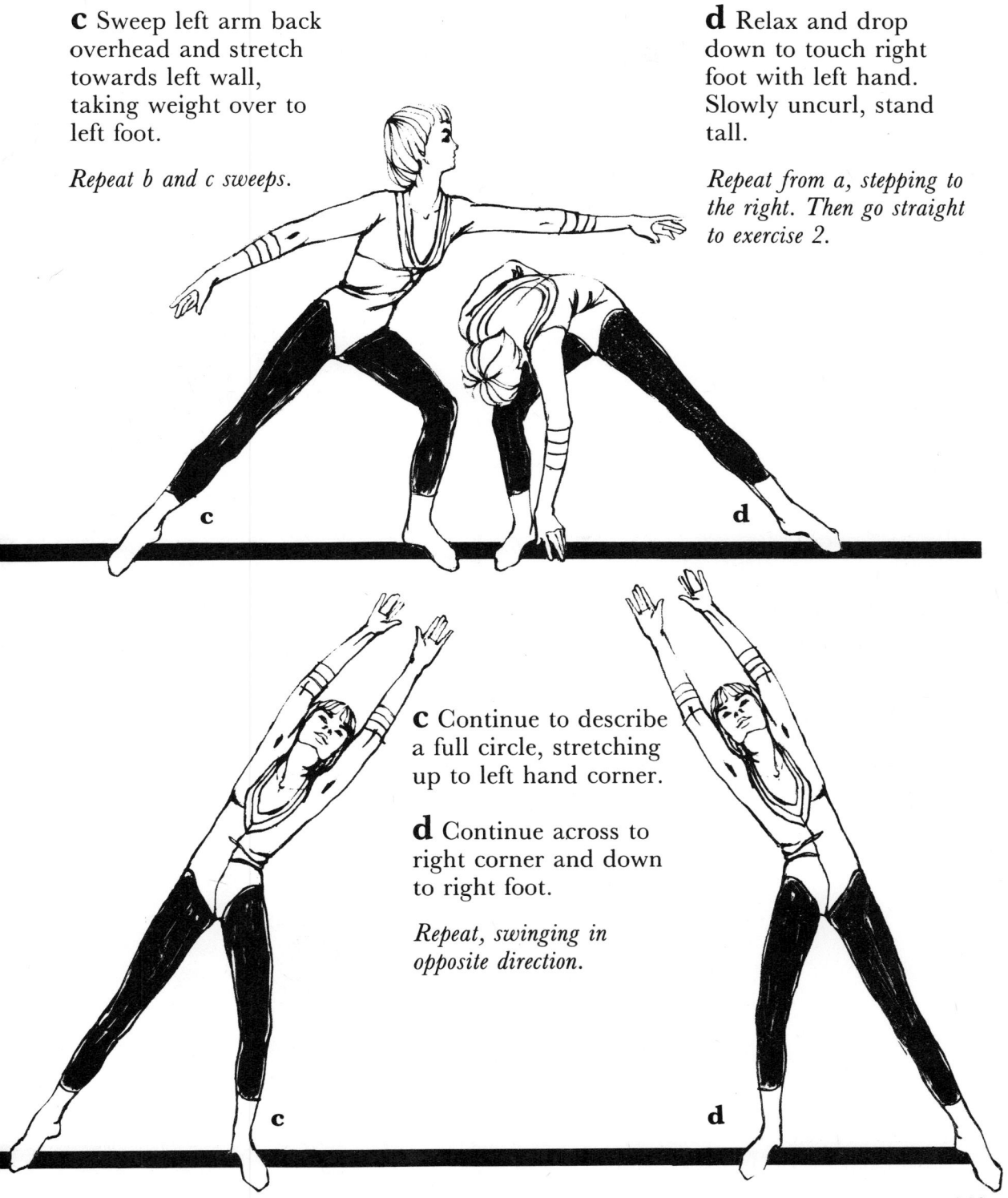

c Continue to describe a full circle, stretching up to left hand corner.

d Continue across to right corner and down to right foot.

Repeat, swinging in opposite direction.

3 LIFT AND KICK

A strong lift for abdomen and hips. Avoid if wrists are weak.

a Sit on floor with left knee bent, left foot firmly on floor, right leg stretched, hands at sides.

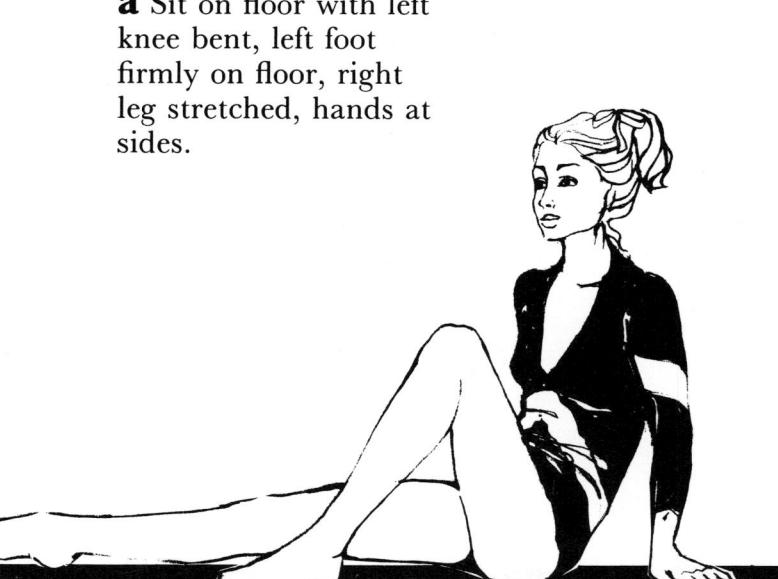

a

4 FLOOR SIDE STRETCH

A 'top to toe' stretch to firm and slim the waistline.

a Sit sideways on floor with left knee bent, right leg straight.

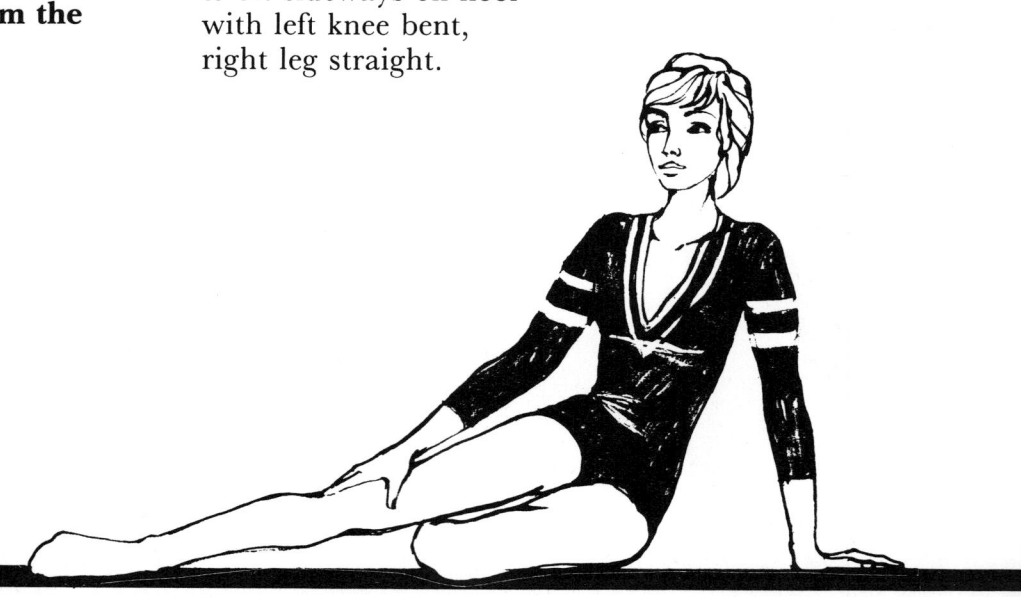

a

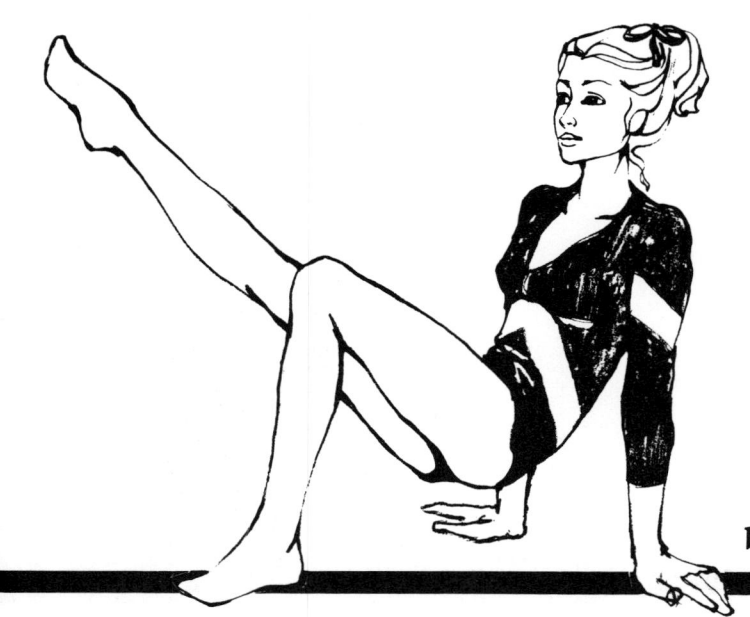

b With weight on hands and left foot, kick with right leg, lifting seat off floor. Lower leg.

Repeat 3 times. Change legs.

b

b With weight on left hand and left knee, lift off the floor, as right arm comes up sideways close to head.

Return to start and repeat on other side.

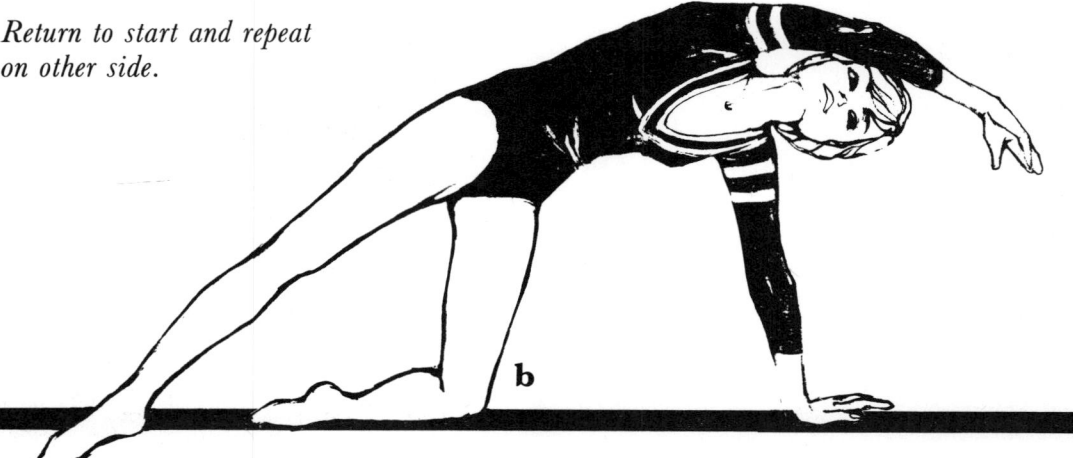

b

5 RELAX AND STRETCH

A sustained stretch to benefit back, chest and shoulders.

a Kneel on left knee, right knee bent with foot flat on floor. Relax over knee to touch floor just beyond toes.

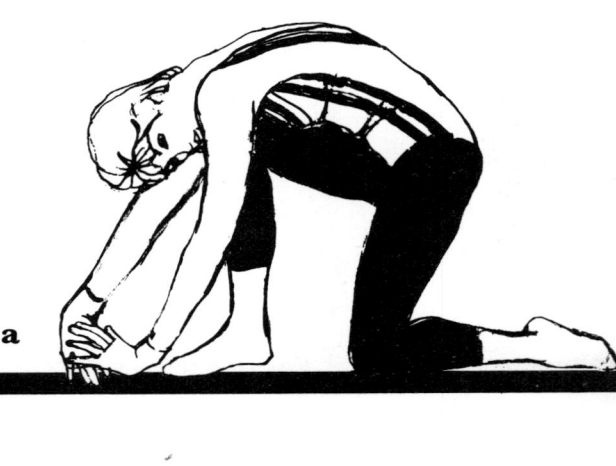

a

6 'UP AND OVER'

Basic waistline side stretch with emphasis on leg muscles.

a Kneel on right knee with left leg stretched out at side. Raise right arm up sideways.

b Curve arm, bending to left.

Repeat, on left knee.

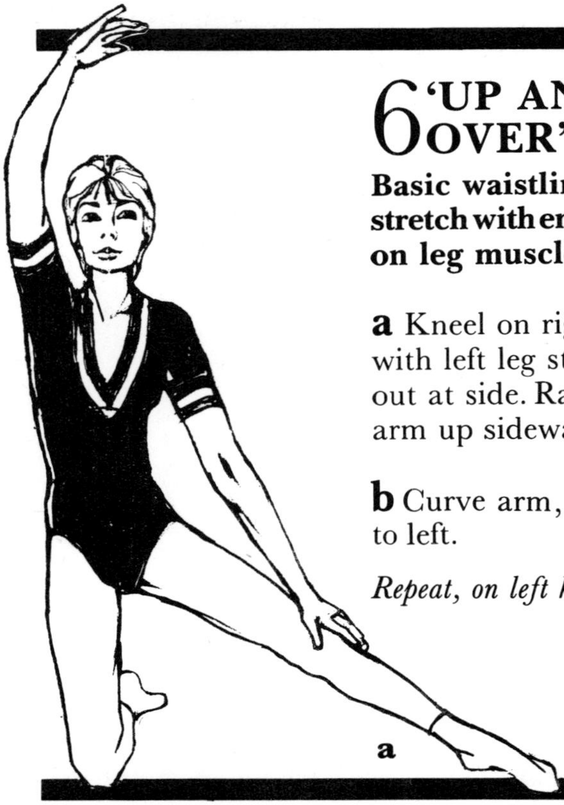

a

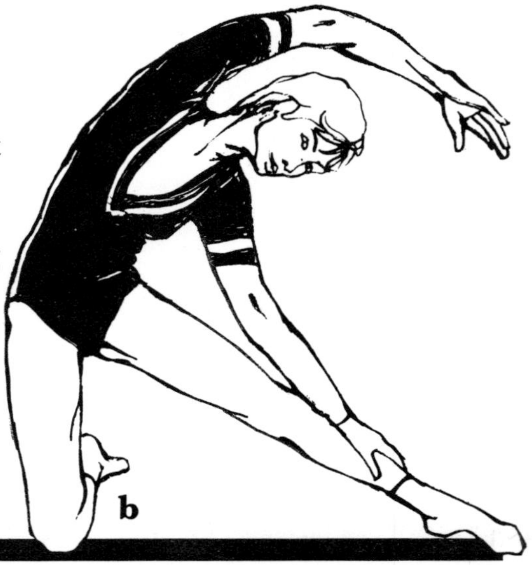

b

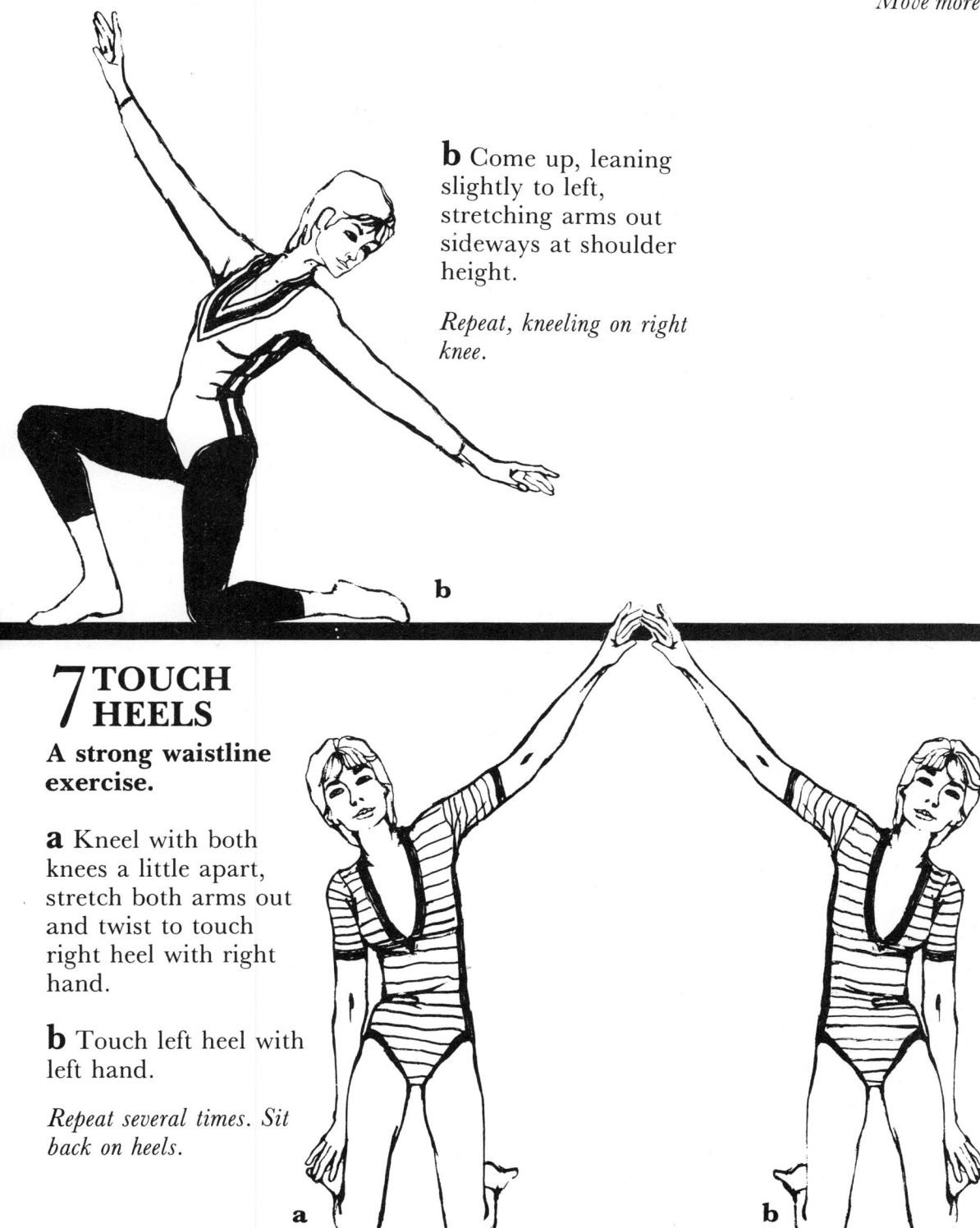

b Come up, leaning slightly to left, stretching arms out sideways at shoulder height.

Repeat, kneeling on right knee.

7 TOUCH HEELS

A strong waistline exercise.

a Kneel with both knees a little apart, stretch both arms out and twist to touch right heel with right hand.

b Touch left heel with left hand.

Repeat several times. Sit back on heels.

147

8 SIDE KICK

A 'stay supple' movement for maximum hip mobility.

a Lie on right side, head resting on arm, left arm overhead.

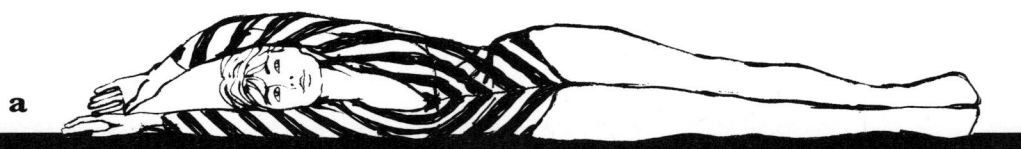

9 SIDE LIFT

To firm the legs, thighs, hips and seat.

a Lie on right side with right arm bent to support head, and left hand placed comfortably in front.

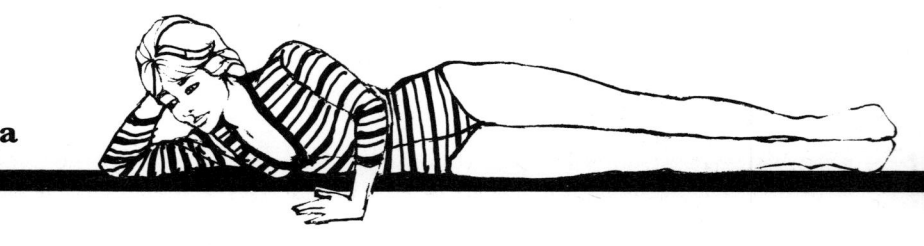

b Lift top leg in high side kick, bringing top arm up to touch foot.

Turn and repeat.

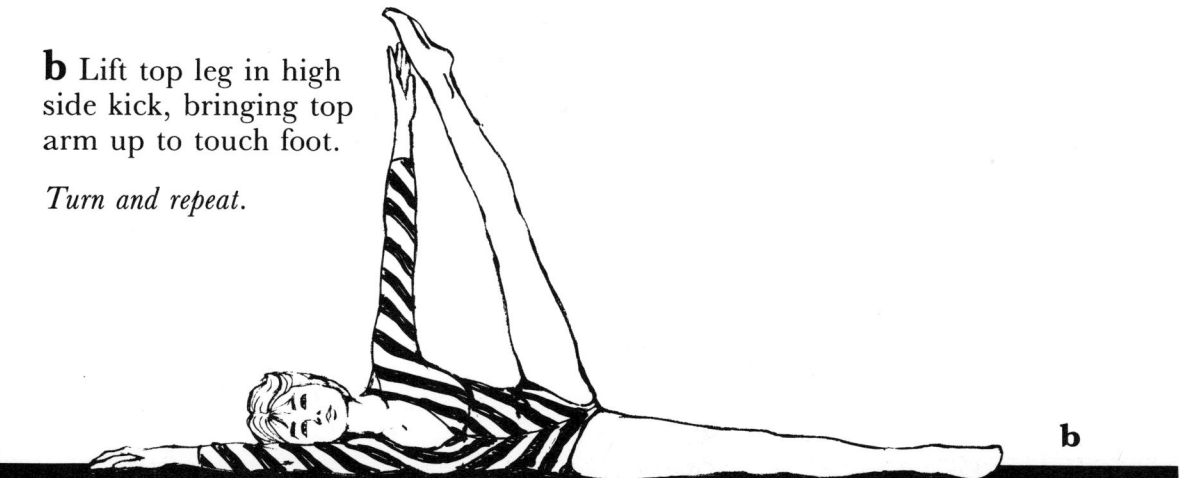

b

b Push down with left hand and raise both legs as high as possible. Lower legs slowly.

Turn and repeat.

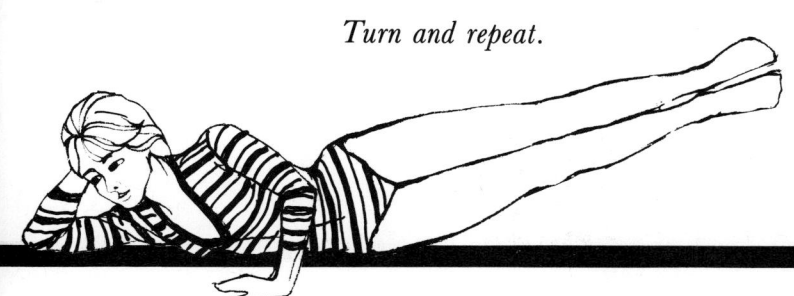

b

149

10 ROLL BACK, TOUCH TOES

To fine down the figure.

a Sit on floor, hands at sides. Roll backwards, bringing knees towards chest.

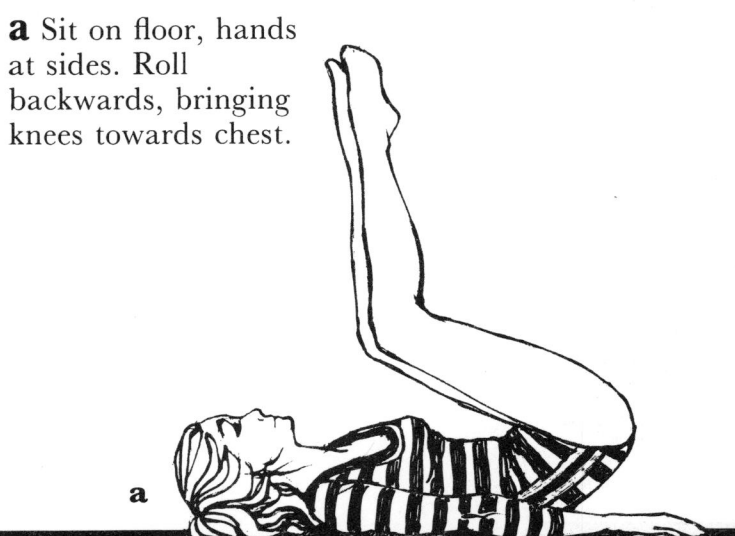

a

11 SHOULDER STAND

An acrobatic exercise for the young and fit; not recommended for anyone with health problems.

a Start from sitting position and roll backwards, bringing up hands to support waist, elbows on floor, stretch legs up towards ceiling.

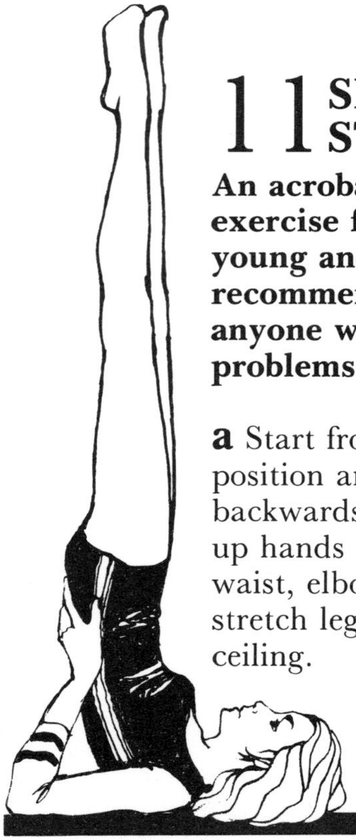

a

b When steady, allow both legs to fall gently overhead.

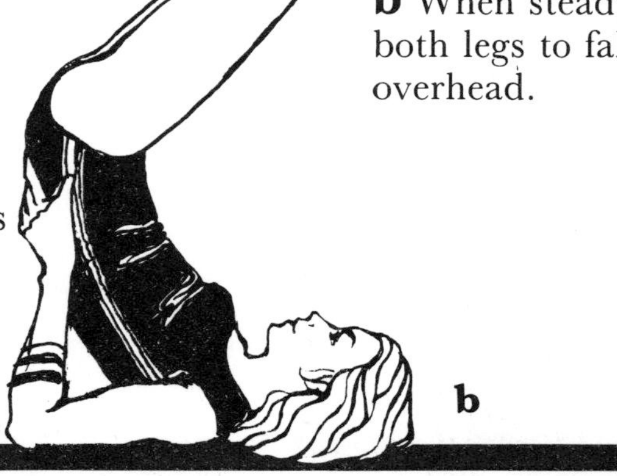

b

b Roll forward immediately and cross ankles.

c Reach forward to touch toes.

Repeat several times, and relax.

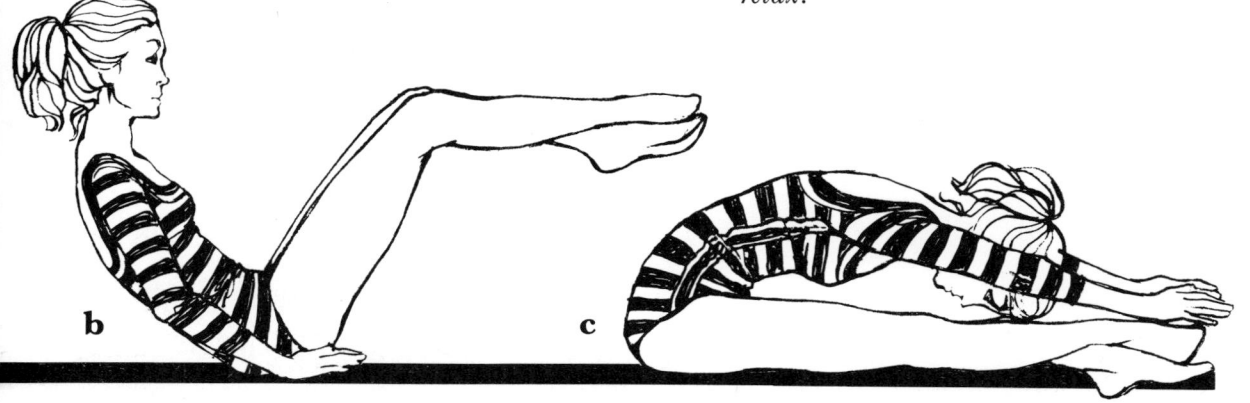

b

c

c In final stage, release hands, toes to floor behind head. Slowly and carefully unroll to lie flat on floor.

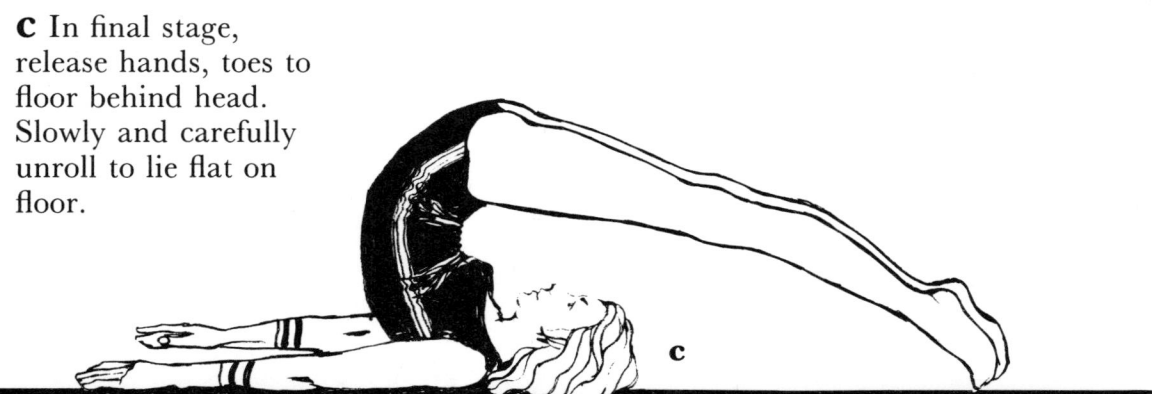

c

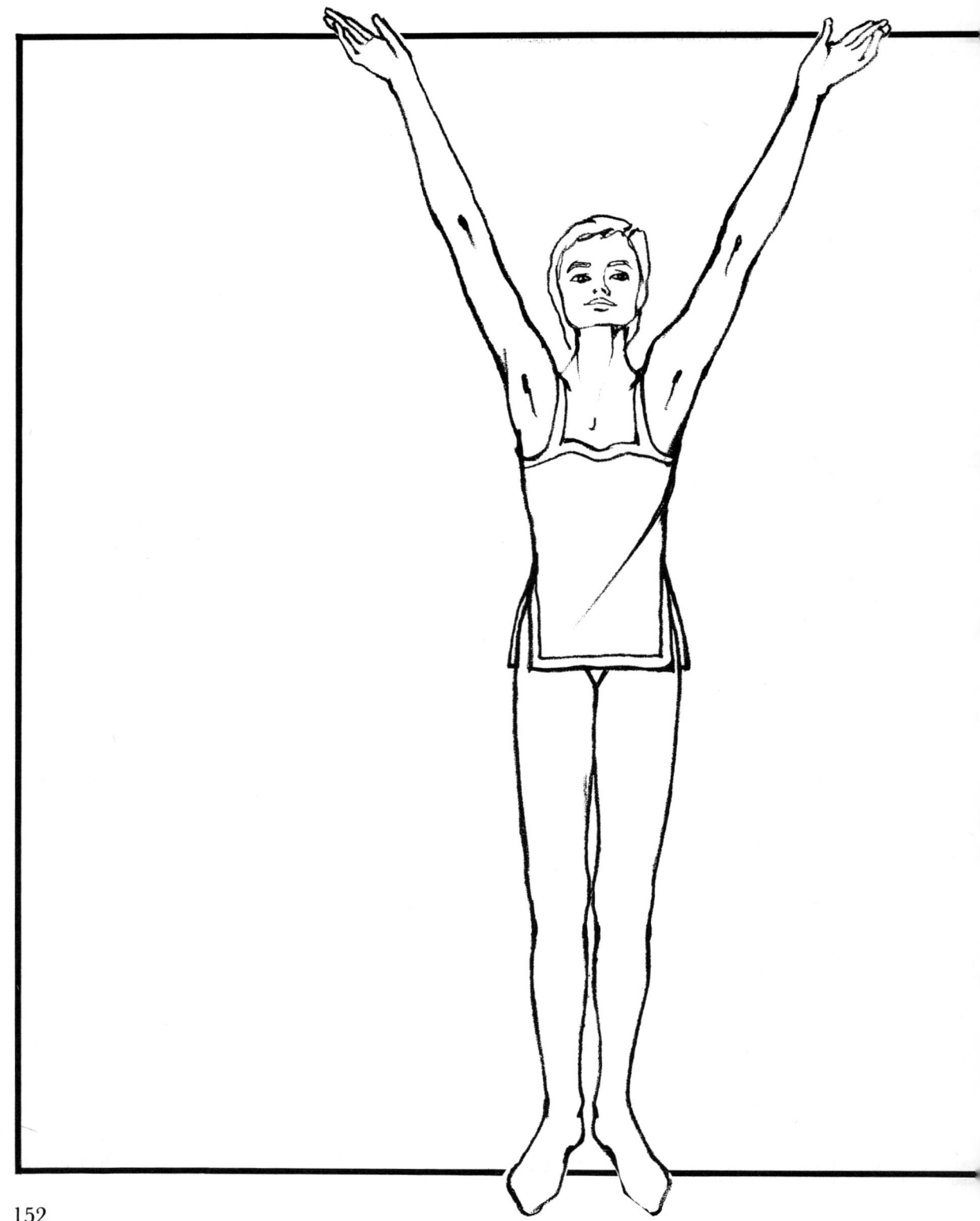

Chapter 16

Morning choice

A two-minute routine

To my mind, a good stretch in the morning is worth two in the afternoon. Later in the day we loosen up, stand straighter and are more mobile, but first thing in the morning is the time we need a lift. Two or three stretches, a swing and a bend are quite enough to take away any stiffness after a night's rest and these exercises are found in the following routine which takes just two minutes to run through. Exercises 1, 2 and 4 (the three ways to stretch upwards) are the most valuable, so try to find time for these. The swing around (3) and the knee bend (5) get the body moving, so do these as well if you have time.

Any stiffness present in hands, feet or shoulders can be greatly helped by the little exercises in Chapters 7 and 18. Shrugging and rolling the shoulders, and bending and stretching legs and feet, all aid mobility and the will to 'get going'.

1 YAWN AND STRETCH

For an early morning lift.

Bend the elbows, stretch up slowly and strongly. Hold for several seconds, lower arms, and repeat.

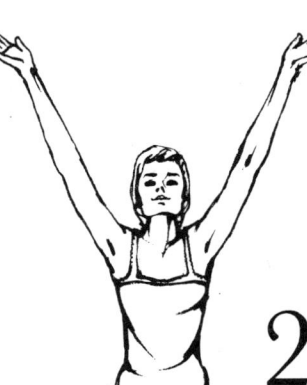

2 CLIMBING CLAPS

A strong stretch for waistline and back muscles.

With feet apart, take arms up sideways. Clap overhead 3 times, getting higher and higher with each clap.

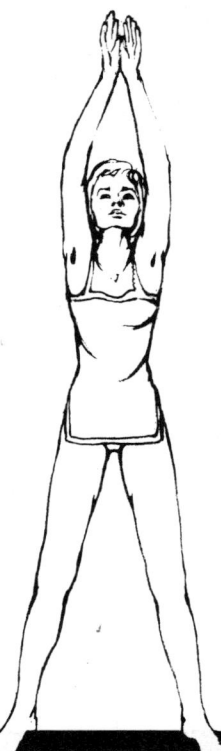

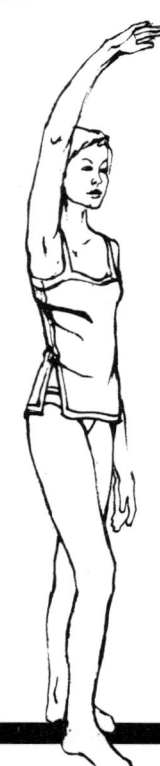

4 BACKSTROKE

To strengthen pectoral muscles, shoulders and upper back.

Circle each arm in turn – forward, up, back and down. (Keep arm close to side of head.)

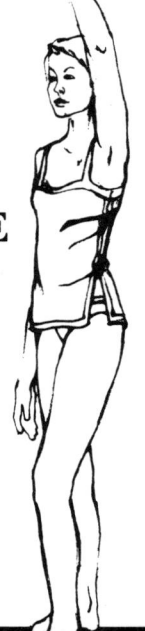

3 SWING AROUND

To lift the chest and slim the waist.

a Feet apart, bend right arm across chest. Keep knees easy.

b Swing arm round to right and return.

Repeat 3 times and change the arm.

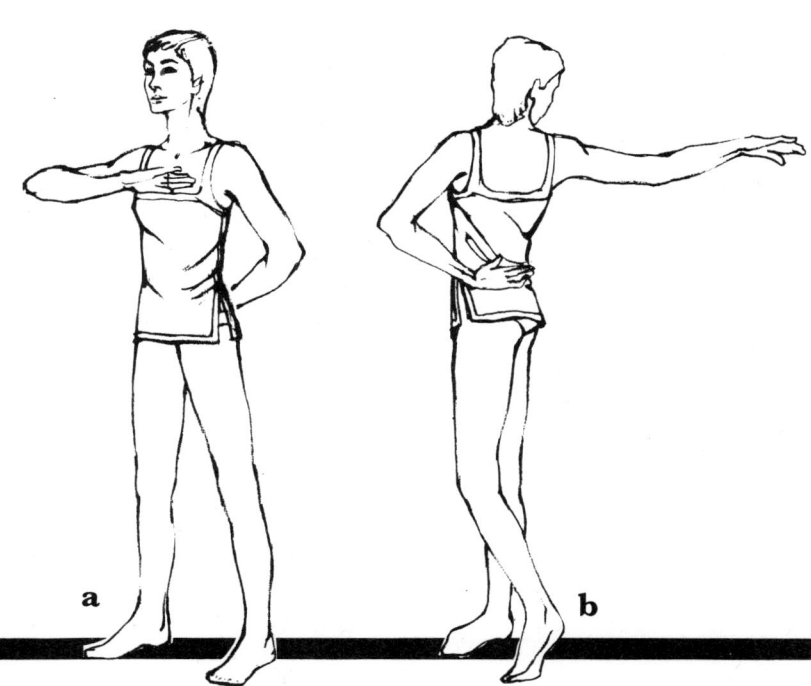

a

b

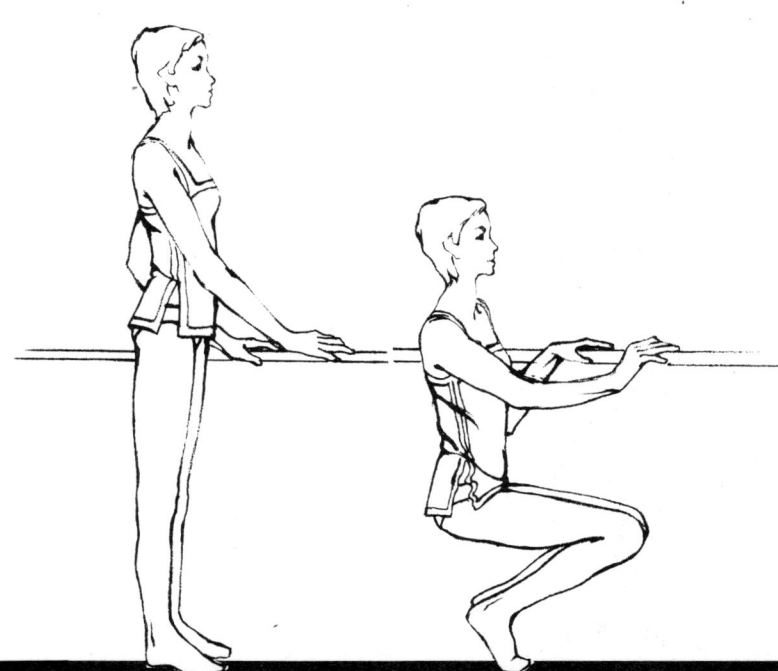

5 DEEP KNEE BEND

To mobilise knees and strengthen legs and thighs.

Well supported, bend both knees deeply, keeping back straight. Come up slowly.

155

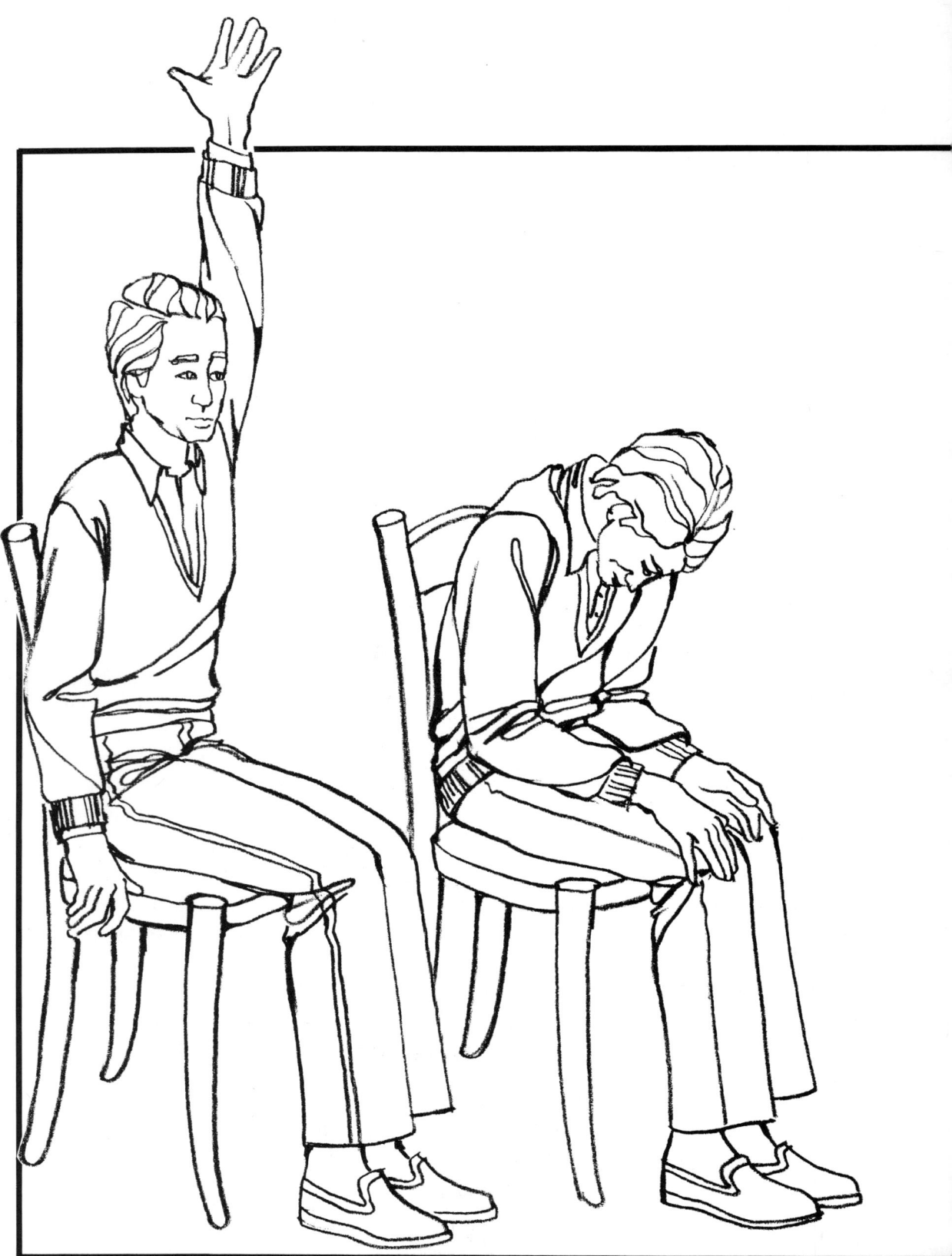

Chapter 17

Muscular relaxation

Movements for the recognition of tension

To suggest exercise as a source of relaxation may sound like a contradiction in terms, but this is not so. By practising these 'stretch and flop' movements, tension becomes instantly recognisable and can be treated at once. The main problem with tension is that we are not always aware that we are tense. We therefore do nothing about it, and the longer tension builds, the harder it is to release.

The drawings in this chapter show the contrast between tension and relaxation very clearly, and by practising the first three exercises, the difference can be felt. Once the feeling of 'flop and let go' becomes automatic, hunched shoulders will drop and tight neck muscles will relax.

In exercises 4 and 5 you will see two positions for a quick recovery from mental and physical exhaustion. For complete relaxation, the recommended position is flat out on the floor. In cases where this is not comfortable, the knees can be drawn up close, relieving any back strain, as in exercise 4. The feet-up position in 5 is a version of the American 'body slant', when the whole body lies on a board which is tipped up at one end. Here, the feet are higher than the head – at a height which will prove both relaxing and refreshing.

1 STRETCH AND LET GO

For the recognition of tension in arms and legs, and the feel of relaxation.

a Sit with feet firmly on floor and stretch right arm strongly. Hold for count of ten.

b Drop arm into lap, and let go.

Repeat with left arm.

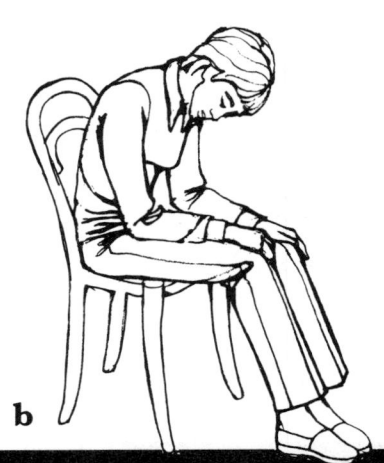

a

b

2 STRETCH AND FLOP

For the contrast of tension and relaxation in the shoulders, neck, arms and upper body.

a Stretch up with both arms for count of ten.

b Flop over knees.

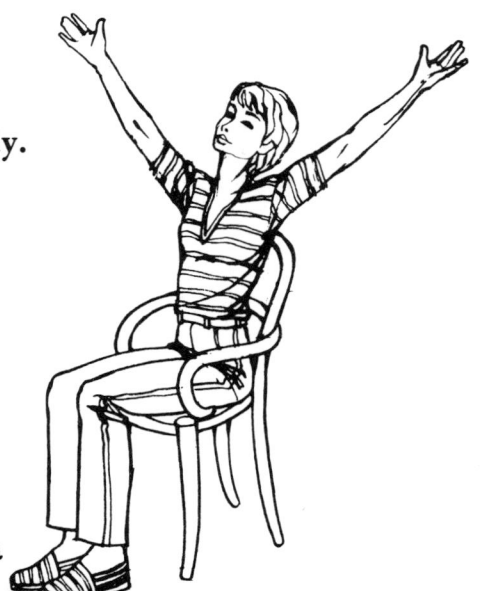

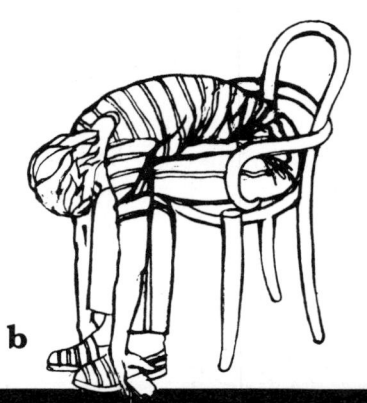

a

b

c Stretch right leg forward strongly. Hold for as long as possible.

d Relax leg and lower foot to floor, and let go.

Repeat with left leg.

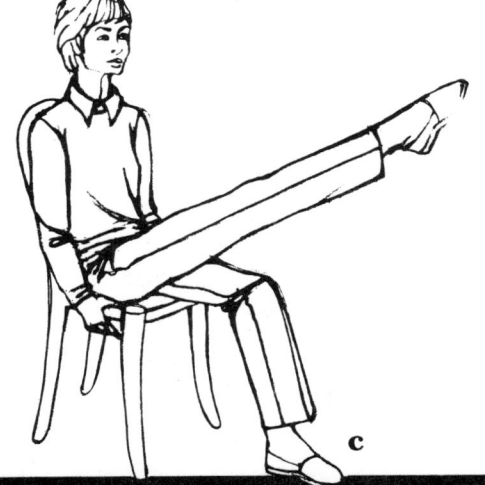

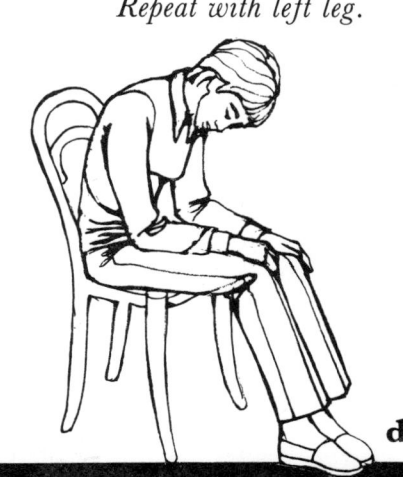

c Stretch up with both arms again.

d Relax.

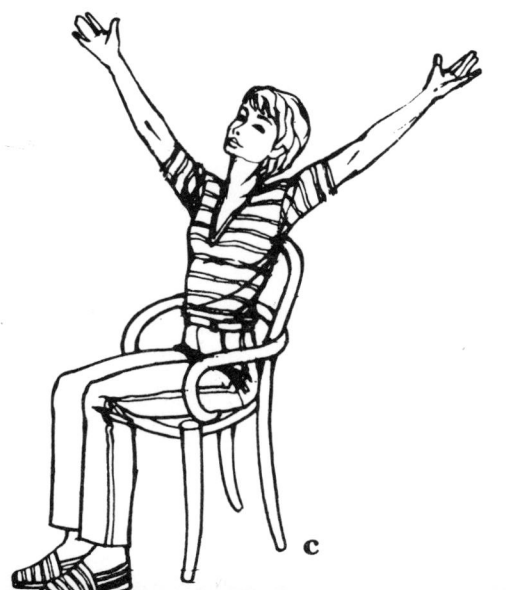

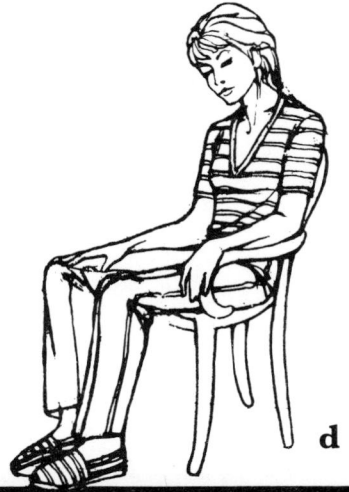

3 PULL UP AND RELAX

A stretch for a lift in the waistline, followed by a feeling of relaxation.

a Stretch right arm up strongly, close to head, and hold. Feel pull in waistline.

b Let the arm drop into lap. Feel muscles relax.

Repeat with left arm.

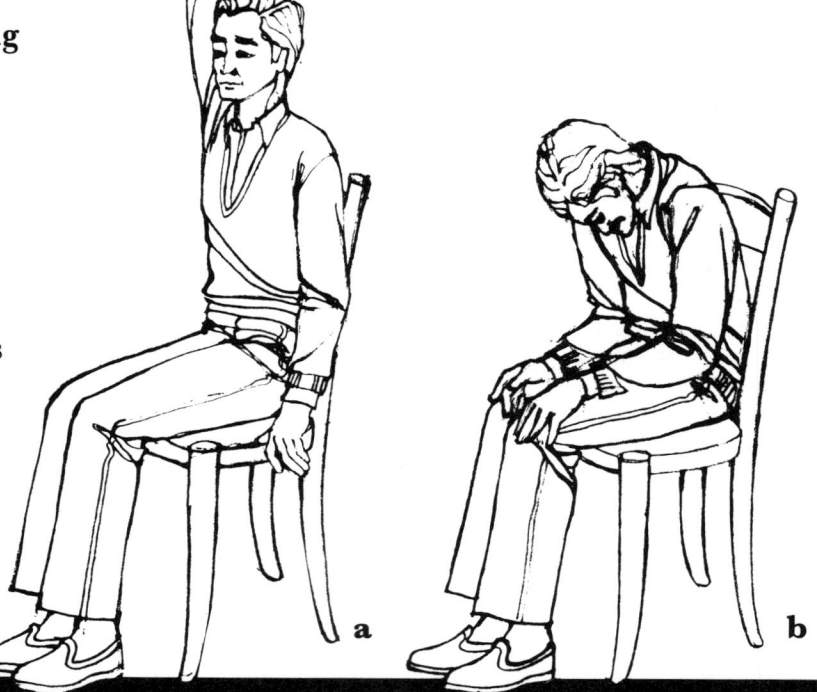

4 KNEES BEND AND RELAX

An alternative position if strain is felt in the back when legs are straight.

Lie flat on floor. Relax back into floor, bend knees at comfortable height.

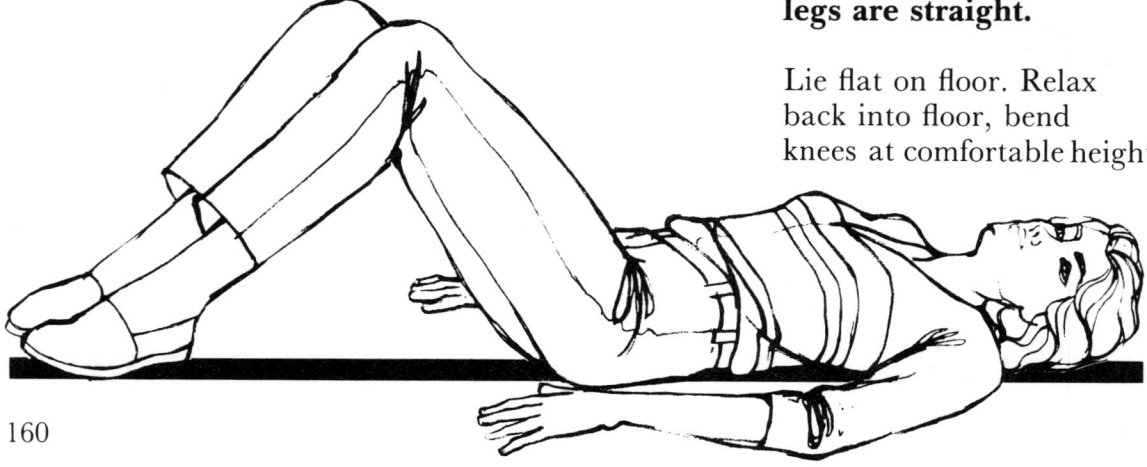

160

5 FEET UP AND RELAX

Feet higher than head to relieve tension and exhaustion.

Lie flat with both feet up on seat of chair.

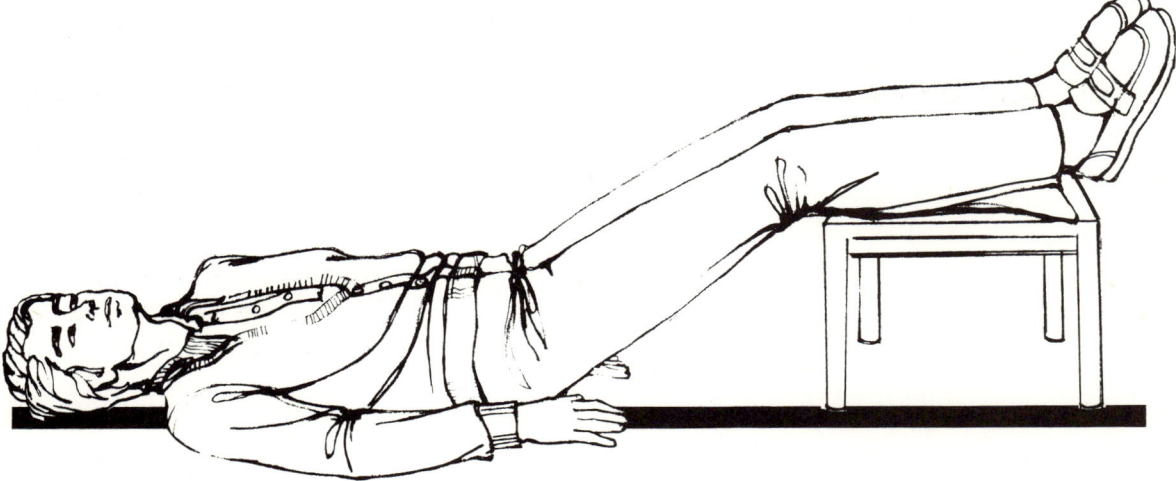

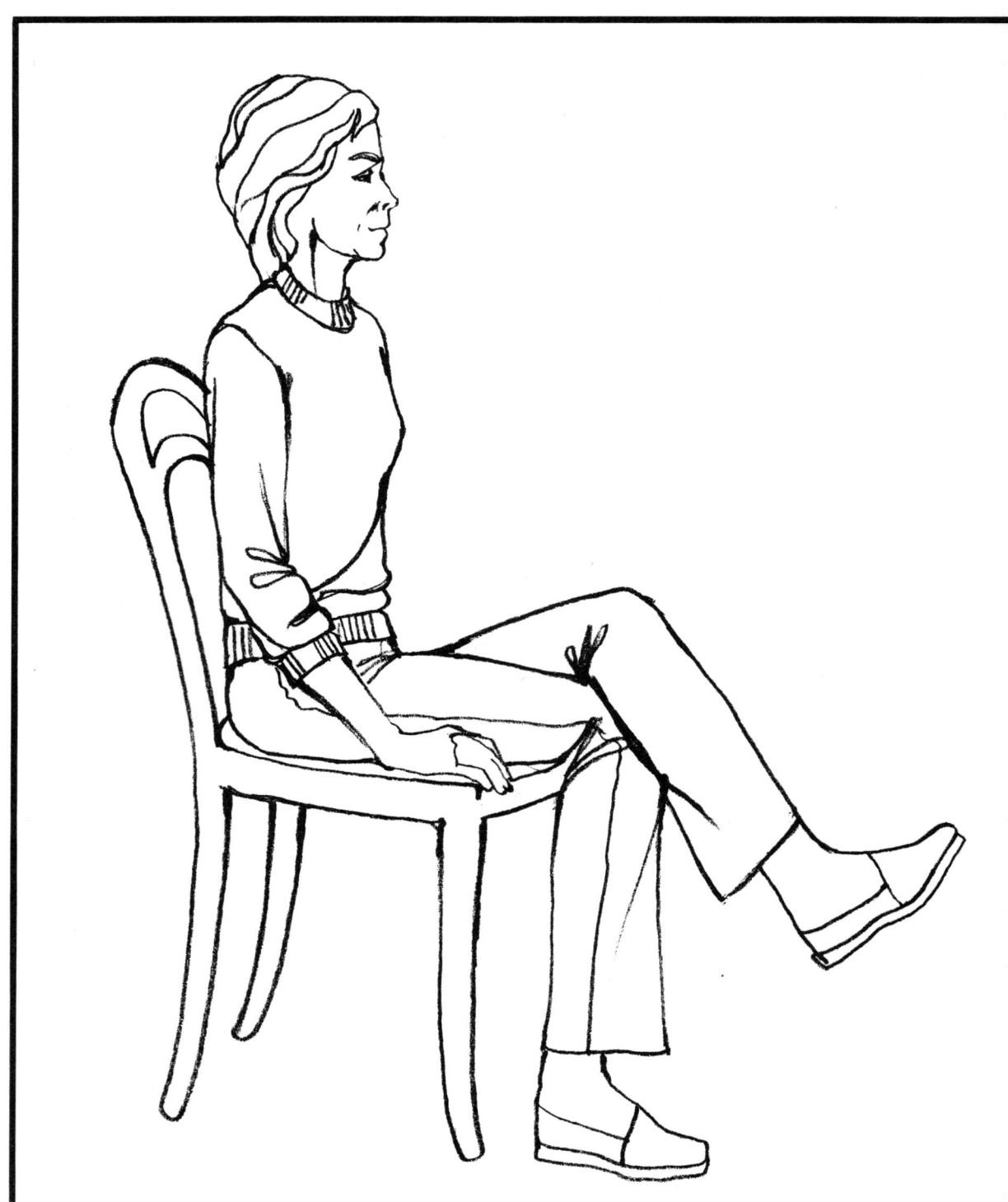

Chapter 18

As young as you feel

Sit and stay supple

Here are six chair exercises which are mainly for mobility. There is nothing static about them, so a firm straight-backed chair is best, and will allow for a greater range of movement. The exercises are a little slower, smaller and more gentle than those in earlier chapters, but this makes them suitable for beginners, and for people who prefer to sit. I have great faith in these exercises, which include foot movements, 'swimming', and the special 'pull in' to strengthen slack stomach muscles.

The elbow swing, exercise 5, is rather like rocking the baby, but it does mobilise shoulders and the upper back. The last one is quite strong for a sitting exercise, but for anyone who wishes to move more, it is worth practising. Its main purpose is to strengthen the abdominal muscles.

'Musical chairs', as these exercises are sometimes called, can be both therapeutic and entertaining at the same time. Many a keep fit leader has taken classes of this type with senior members of various organisations. At home, attractive melodies make the movements more interesting, and records and tapes are available if required. For details, see Chapter 20.

1 TOES UP, TOES DOWN

To give greater mobility to the feet.

a Sit well back in chair, cross right leg over left and move toes up and down 7 times. Change legs on 8, and repeat.

b With legs crossed, circle foot from the ankle 7 times. Change legs on 8, and repeat.

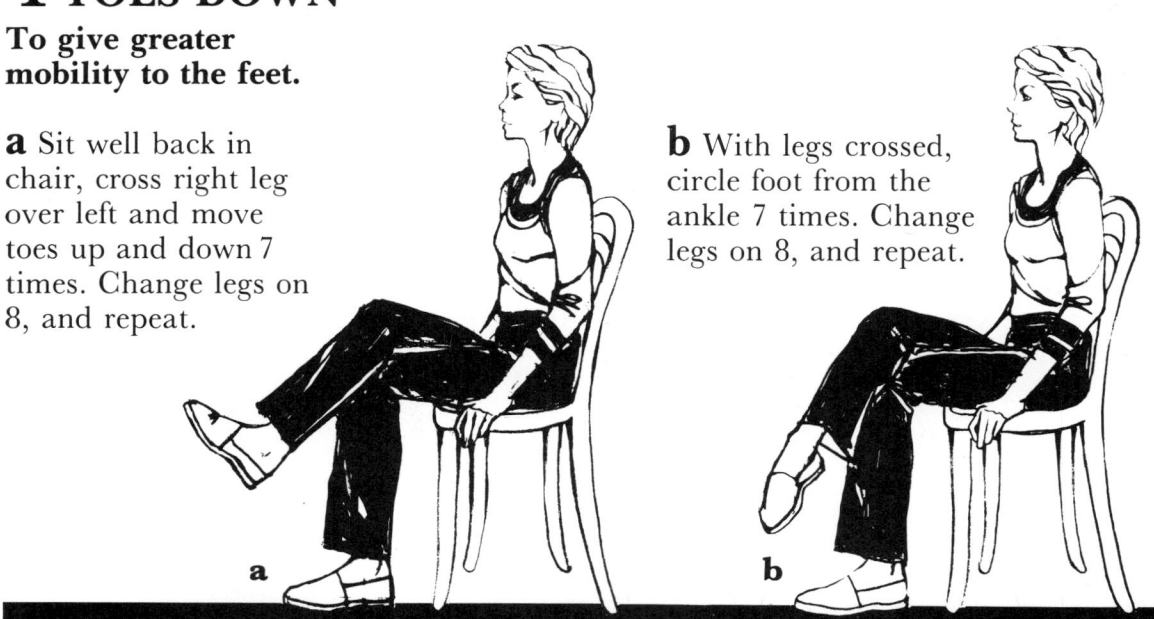

3 REACH OUT AND SWIM

To give a lift to the chest and to improve posture.

a Sit well forward in chair and bring elbows in close, hands side by side. Stretch one leg.

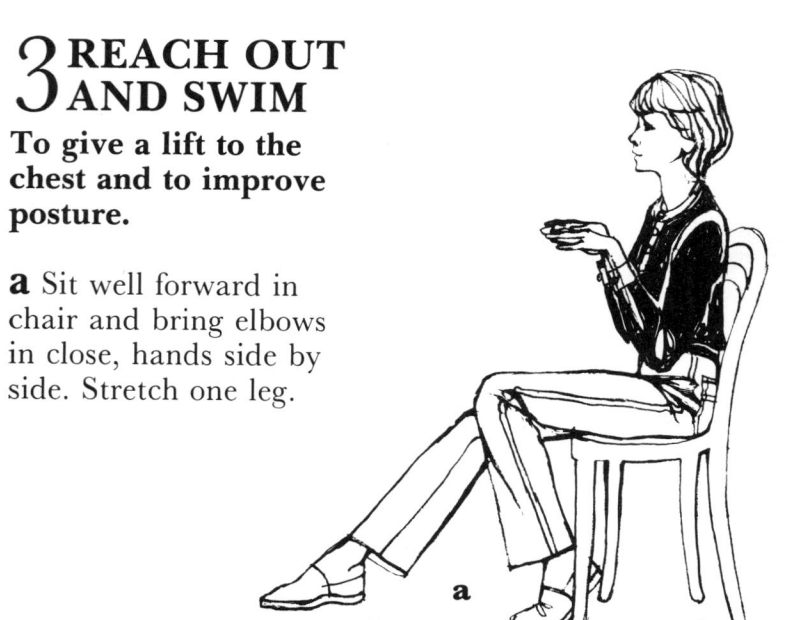

2 HEEL TAP AND KNEE LIFT

To strengthen instep, ankles, calves, and for easy knees.

a Keeping toes on the floor, raise heels. Tap heels gently on floor 7 times, rest on 8. Rest for further 8 counts, and repeat.

b Lift right knee and clasp to support. Stretch leg forward, bend knee, release and put foot to floor.

Repeat with left knee.

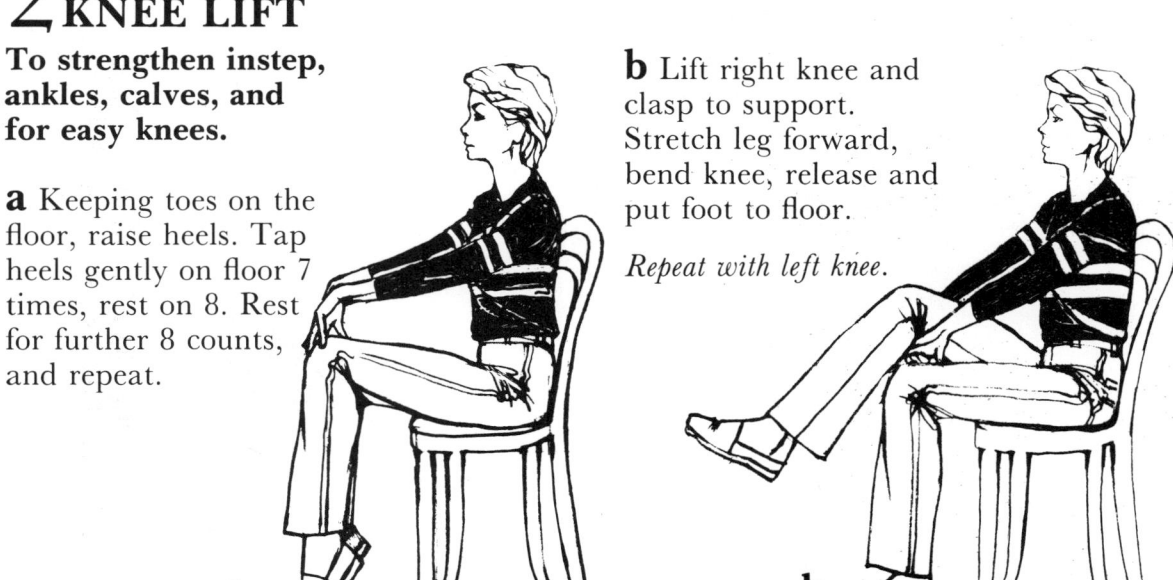

b Reach forward, stretching both arms as in breast-stroke.

c Pull arms back strongly to stretch sideways at shoulder height.

Repeat several times, and relax.

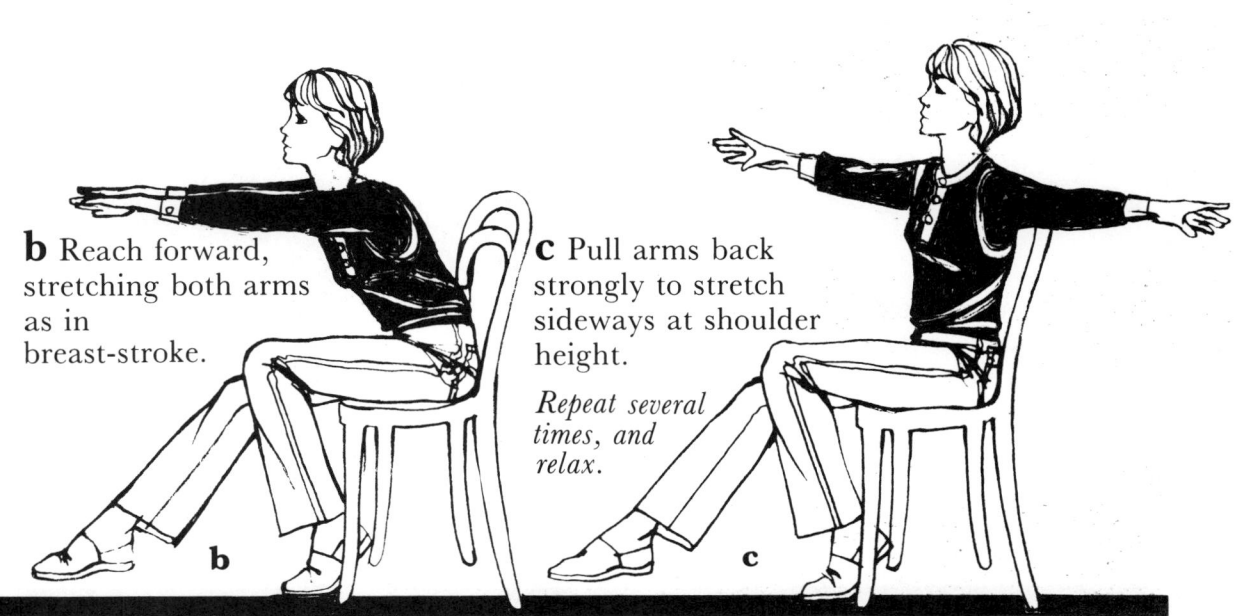

4 PULL IN, LET GO

To strengthen stomach muscles.

Sit tall and well back in chair. With both hands on stomach muscles, pull in towards spine and then let go.

Repeat more strongly, and relax.

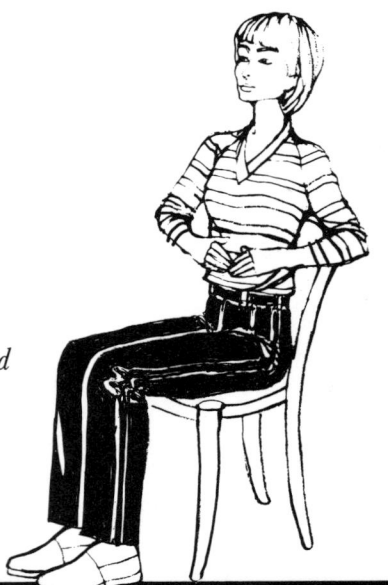

5 ELBOW SWING

To mobilise chest, shoulders and upper back.

a Bend elbows, fists lightly touching. Swing both elbows high to right.

b Swing both elbows across chest to left, moving shoulders as much as possible.

Swing to right and repeat.

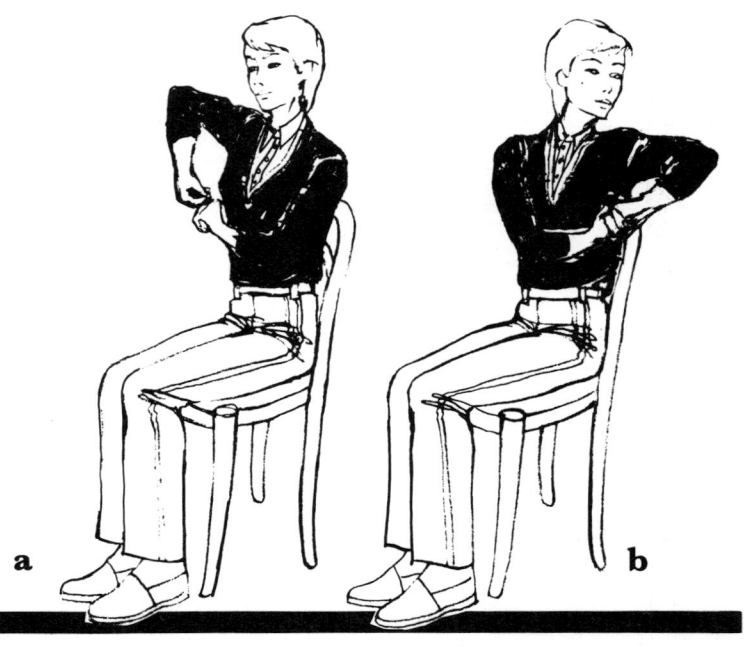

a   b

6 STRETCH AND RELAX

A progression on exercise 4, to strengthen abdominal muscles.

a Bend forward and sideways, reaching down to the floor with right hand, left arm stretched.

b Return to good sitting position.

c Bend forward and reach down with left hand, right arm stretched. Sit up, sit tall.

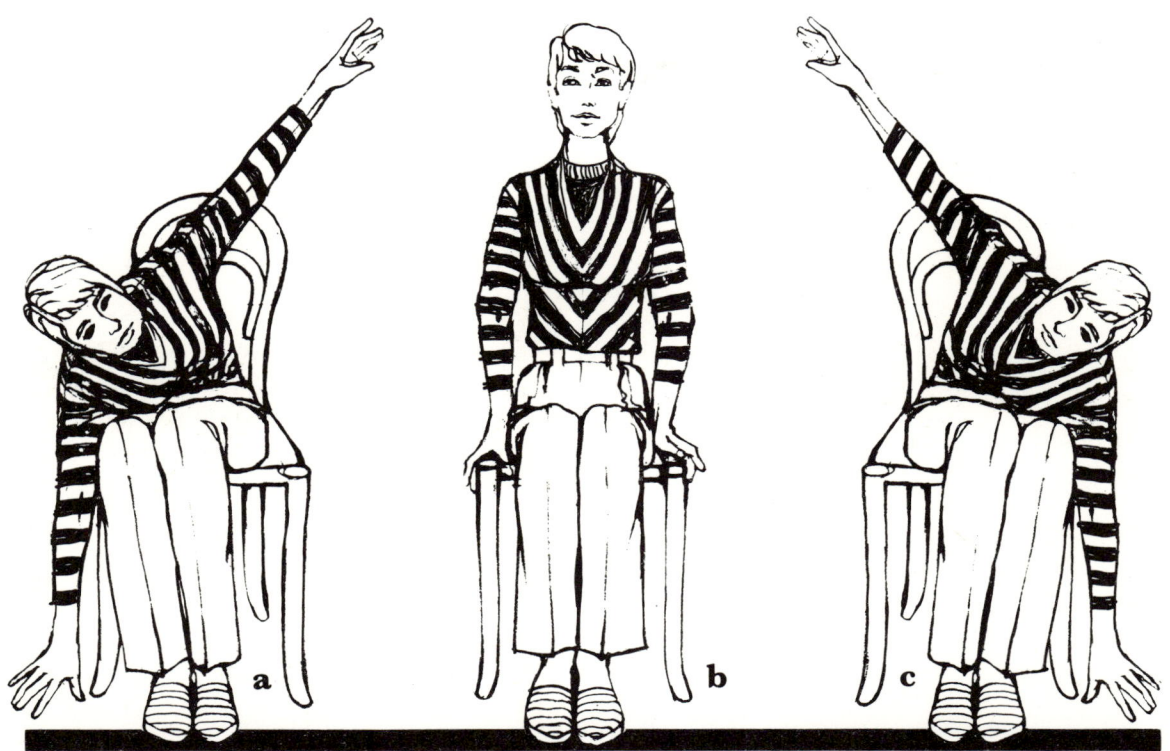

Chapter 19

The
Keep Fit Association
and Sports Centres

We are fortunate today because we have all types of movement and sport available to us; the choice is wide and standards very high. As a founder and life member of the Keep Fit Association, it has been my privilege to see great changes and much progress in this field. Before the war a number of us were teaching keep fit in many parts of the country. Wonderful work was done by Norah Reed in the North of England, and other leaders were very busy indeed in the South.

My own contribution to the keep fit movement was an industrial keep fit organisation, with classes in Middlesex, Hertfordshire and Essex. Much help was given by the Central Council of Recreation, their senior technical advisors attending my 5,000-strong keep fit pageants.

The League of Health and Beauty had a tremendously large membership and people flocked to Wembley to watch their demonstrations.

Eventually, those of us who were working either privately or for the education authorities came together to form the Keep Fit Association, which has gone from strength to strength during the last twenty-seven years. Strong backing came from the BBC with the presentation of my television and radio programmes, and now there is a keep fit class in practically every city, town and village in Great Britain. Fourteen thousand people watch the two annual demonstrations at the Albert Hall, and more than 30,000 are members of the Association.

The Keep Fit Association was formed in 1956 to bring together the various regional and local associations. Its first task was to consolidate the great variety of work carried out under the name of keep fit, and then to establish a common standard for training its teachers which would be acceptable, not only to its members, but to the many local authorities throughout the country.

To achieve this the KFA:

Co-operates closely with local Education Authorities, the Sports Council, and other associations representing the community, for example the Department of Health and Social Security.

Organises conferences and training courses for members who are leaders, trainers or pianists.

Arranges an annual national festival, and an Annual General Meeting within a large national festival.

Plans rallies, demonstrations and social events.

Publishes a national magazine, diary, training syllabus and other training material.

Teachers' Award

In 1974, following the success of the national Leaders' Award, a new Teachers' Award was established to provide members with two stages of assessment. Training courses to prepare candidates are held regionally, when and where there is sufficient demand.

How the KFA can help you

The Keep Fit Association exists primarily to promote keep fit classes for women. Its aims are:

To promote physical and mental well-being.

To help women to move with poise and grace.

To provide enjoyment and companionship.

The KFA has pride in its trained teachers who know their subject and methods of teaching. Keep fit is a vital activity which combines music and exercise. Today's leaders create an exciting, modern image and use cassettes, tapes, and the piano to provide lively music. Keep fit is not an endurance test but teachers are aware of the need to provide a good measure of strong, rapid work which stimulates circulation and increases stamina. There is a place for everyone, no matter of what age, to join in an activity which is well-balanced and full of contrasts. It helps class members to lose inches, to tone up muscles and to become more shapely. Members are encouraged to eat sensibly and thus to become and to stay slim.

Membership

The Association relies on individual subscriptions from all those who enjoy and benefit from their local keep fit classes, and from others who wish to show their support of the Association's activities.

For information on membership of your local Keep Fit Association and keep fit class, write for an application form to:

**The National Secretary,
Keep Fit Association,
16 Upper Woburn Place,
London WC1H 0QG.**

Keep fit rallies

Wherever there are keep fit classes you can be sure that sooner or later a rally will be organised. Rallies are very popular events and girls and women of all ages attend. A tremendous number of them are held within the Keep Fit Association itself, and my organisers run many others in conjunction with local Associations.

A large hall, ballroom or seaside pavilion is booked months ahead for a Saturday or Sunday afternoon. The rally lasts from 2 p.m. until 5 p.m., with a 45-minute break for demonstrations. The numbers of participants vary, but there are seldom less than seven or eight hundred people, all dressed in leotards and generating a marvellous atmosphere.

The programme is as varied as possible to suit everyone – there are warm-ups, floor exercises, and flowing movements for balance and poise interspersed with dance routines. The current choice is for dance mobility, movements to disco rhythm or to tunes high in the charts, and the pace quickens until it is time to finish.

Sports Centres

There is one Sports Centre in particular that I would like to tell you about, and that is the Alton Sports Centre in Hampshire. Similar facilities exist in many other centres throughout the country. I can, however, speak about Alton at first hand as I have taken Keep Fit Rallies there. It is managed by Robert Tedder, a splendid man, an organiser *par excellence*, with a great deal of enthusiasm and personal charm. He would be the first to say how much he owes the success of the Centre to his excellent staff. For them no hours of the day are too long.

People of all ages flock to the Alton Sports Centre, as the accent is not only on training for a specific sport but on the needs of the whole family. Much emphasis is laid upon recreation, meaning the re-creation of bodily health, and the whole place is alive with the spirit of enjoyment and fun. Activities range from games for children to sports and slightly less energetic activities for older people. Active leisure is the operative word, including a very busy and popular social side.

Special events are planned for the physically handicapped and suitable facilities are available. A coaching and instruction scheme for mentally handicapped people was started recently – with great success.

Other facilities include swimming pools, a sauna suite, a projectile fitness room and fitness testing centre, plus a very large activity hall. The Centre caters for the following activities:

Archery	Fencing	Netball
Badminton	Fitness Training	Shooting
(7 courts)	Keep Fit Classes	Swimming
Basketball	Football	Squash
Bowls (3 rinks)	Golf	Table Tennis
Boxing	Gymnastics	(7 tables)
Canoeing	Hockey	Tennis
Climbing	Judo	Trampoline
Country Dancing	Karate	Volleyball
Cricket (2 nets)	Modern Ballroom Dancing	Weight Training

Information on the Sports Centres in your area is available at public libraries. Alternatively, contact your regional office of the Sports Council or write to:

**The Sports Council,
16 Upper Woburn Place,
London WC1H 0QP.**

Chapter 20

Information

Keep Fit with Eileen Fowler
'Meet Eileen Fowler' rallies are arranged from time to time throughout the country. All enquiries should be addressed to The Secretary, 'Glebe', Mill Lane, Horndon-on-the-Hill, Essex.

Keep fit music and instruction
To assist anyone wishing to practise the exercises contained in Chapters 9, 10, 11, 12, 13 and 18 to specially arranged music and instruction, records and tapes are available (see opposite).

These keep fit records have been used to start up keep fit groups in rural areas as in the initial stages it is not always possible to find an experienced leader or pianist. When starting a group among friends or fellow workers it is advisable to learn the basic movements carefully yourself before demonstrating them 'in class' to the record. In this way, all members of the group can get the utmost benefit from the recorded routines. If possible, a leader should be chosen and encouraged to take training as soon as possible. The Keep Fit Association or local Education Office will advise.

Keep fit records and cassettes

Family Keep Fit	REC 174 (Stereo)
Enjoy Your Slimming	REC 284
	Cassette ZCM 284
Slim to Rhythm	REC 132 (Stereo)
Dance and Keep Fit	REC 382
	Cassette ZCM 382
As Young As You Feel	REC 195 (Stereo)
	Cassette MRM 007

All records and cassettes carry a BBC label.

Training
Full particulars of leadership training and local keep fit classes may be obtained from:

**The Keep Fit Association,
16 Upper Woburn Place,
London WC1H 0QP.**

For leadership training and local keep fit classes run by the Education Authority, apply to your local Education Office.

Sport for all
For particulars of coaching holidays in a variety of indoor and outdoor activities, Sports Centres and all keep fit facilities, apply to:

**The Sports Council,
16 Upper Woburn Place,
London WC1H 0QP.**